Study Guide to Accompany

POTTER/PERRY

Canadian Fundamentals of Nursing

6th edition

Geralyn Ochs, RN, AGACNP-BC, ACNP-BC, ANP-BC
Associate Professor of Nursing
Coordinator of the Adult Gerontological Acute Care Nurse Practitioner Program
St. Louis University School of Nursing
St. Louis, Missouri

Joyce Engel, RN, PhD
Associate Professor
Department of Nursing
Brock University
St. Catharines, Ontario

Kerry Shoalts, RN, BScN, MEd(c)
Nursing Lab Coordinator
Department of Nursing
Brock University
St. Catharines, Ontario

ELSEVIER

Keeley D

ELSEVIER

Copyright © 2019 Elsevier Canada, a division of Reed Elsevier Canada, Ltd.

This adaptation of the *Study Guide for Fundamentals of Nursing*, 9th edition, by Geralyn Ochs is published by arrangement with Elsevier Inc. ISBN 978-0-323-39644-8 (softcover). Copyright © 2017, Elsevier Inc. All Rights Reserved. Previous editions copyrighted 2013, 2009, 2005, 2001, 1997, 1993, 1989, and 1985.

All rights reserved. No part of this publication may be reproduced or transmitted in any form or by any means, electronic or mechanical, including photocopy, recording, or any information storage and retrieval system, without permission in writing from the publisher. Reproducing passages from this book without such written permission is an infringement of copyright law.

Requests for permission to make copies of any part of the work should be mailed to: College Licensing Officer, access ©, 1 Yonge Street, Suite 1900, Toronto, ON, M5E 1E5. Fax: (416) 868-1621. All other inquiries should be directed to the publisher.

Every reasonable effort has been made to acquire permission for copyright material used in this text, and to acknowledge all such indebtedness accurately. Any errors and omissions called to the publisher's attention will be corrected in future printings.

Notice

Knowledge and best practice in this field are constantly changing. As new research and expertise broaden our knowledge, changes in practice, treatment, and drug therapy may become necessary.

Practitioners and researchers must always rely on their own experience and knowledge in evaluating and using any information, methods, compounds, or experiments described herein. In using such information or methods they should be mindful of their own safety and the safety of others, including parties for whom they have a professional responsibility.

With respect to any drug or pharmaceutical products identified, readers are advised to check the most current information provided (i) on procedures featured or (ii) by the manufacturer of each product to be administered, to verify the recommended dose or formula, the method and duration of administration, and contraindications. It is the responsibility of practitioners, relying on their own experience and knowledge of their patients, to make diagnoses, to determine dosages and the best treatment for each individual patient, and to take all appropriate safety precautions.

To the fullest extent of the law, neither the Publisher nor the authors, contributors, or editors assume any liability for any injury and/or damage to persons or property as a matter of products liability, negligence or otherwise, or from any use or operation of any methods, products, instructions, or ideas contained in the material herein.

The Publisher

Library and Archives Canada Cataloguing in Publication

Ochs, Geralyn, author

Study guide to accompany Potter/Perry Canadian fundamentals of nursing, 6th edition / Geralyn Ochs, RN, AGACNP-BC, ACNP-BC, ANP-BC, Associate Professor of Nursing, Coordinator of the Adult Gerontological Acute Care Nurse Practitioner Program, St. Louis University School of Nursing, St. Louis, Missouri, Joyce Engel, RN, PhD, Associate Professor, Department of Nursing, Brock University, St. Catharines, Ontario, Kerry Shoalts, RN, BScN, Nursing Lab Coordinator, Department of Nursing, Brock University, St. Catharines, Ontario.

ISBN 978-1-77172-126-4 (softcover)

1. Nursing--Problems, exercises, etc. 2. Nursing--Canada--Problems, exercises, etc. I. Engel, Joyce, author II. Shoalts, Kerry, author III. Title.

RT41.P68 2018 Suppl. 610.73 C2017-906577-7

VP Medical and Canadian Education: Madelene J. Hyde
Content Strategist (Acquisitions): Roberta A. Spinosa-Millman
Content Development Manager: Lisa Newton
Content Development Specialist: Martina van de Velde
Publishing Services Manager: Deepthi Unni
Senior Project Manager: Umarani Natarajan
Typesetting and Assembly: TNQ Books and Journals Pvt Ltd, India

Ebook ISBN: 978-1-77172-124-0

Elsevier Canada
420 Main Street East, Suite 636, Milton, ON, Canada L9T 5G3
Phone: 416-644-7053

Last digit is the print number: 9 8 7 6 5 4 3

ISBN: 978-1-77172-126-4

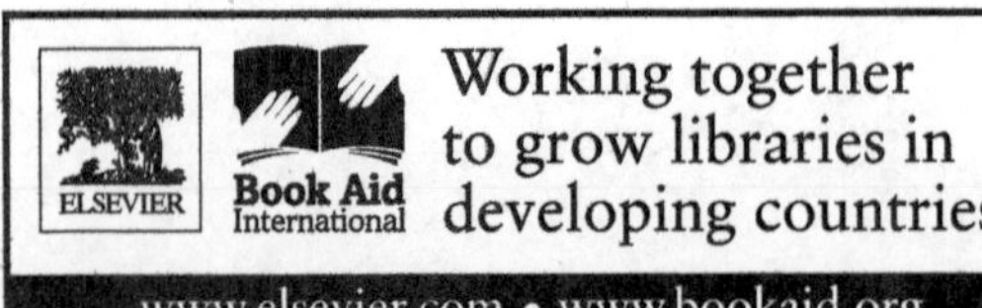

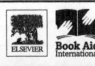

Contents

Introduction, v

UNIT ONE Health and Health Care in Canada
1 Health and Wellness, 1
2 The Canadian Health Care Delivery System, **4**
3 The Development of Nursing in Canada, **7**
4 Community Health Nursing Practice, **10**

UNIT TWO Foundations of Nursing Practice
5 Theoretical Foundations of Nursing Practice, **14**
6 Evidence-Informed Practice, **17**
7 Nursing Values and Ethics, **20**
8 Legal Implications in Nursing Practice, **23**
9 Global Health, **27**
10 Indigenous Health, **30**
11 Nursing Leadership, Management, and Collaborative Practice, **33**

UNIT THREE Approaches to Nursing Care
12 Critical Thinking in Nursing Practice, **36**
13 Nursing Assessment, Diagnosis, and Planning, **39**
14 Implementing and Evaluating Nursing Care, **43**
15 Documenting and Reporting, **46**
16 Nursing Informatics and Canadian Nursing Practice, **50**

UNIT FOUR Working with Patients and Families
17 Communication and Relational Practice, **53**
18 Patient-Centred Care: Interprofessional Collaborative Practice, **59**
19 Family Nursing, **62**
20 Patient Education, **66**

UNIT FIVE Caring Throughout the Lifespan
21 Developmental Theories, **71**
22 Conception Through Adolescence, **76**
23 Young to Middle Adulthood, **84**
24 Older Persons, **88**
25 The Experience of Loss, Death, and Grief, **93**

UNIT SIX Psychosocial Considerations
26 Self-Concept, **97**
27 Sexuality, **102**
28 Spirituality in Health and Health Care, **107**
29 Stress and Adaptation, **111**

UNIT SEVEN Scientific Basis for Nursing Practice
30 Vital Signs, **116**
31 Pain Assessment and Management, **124**
32 Health Assessment and Physical Examination, **133**

Copyright © 2019 Elsevier Canada, a division of Reed Elsevier Canada, Ltd.

33 Infection Control, **143**
34 Medication Administration, **150**
35 Complementary and Alternative Approaches in Health Care, **164**

UNIT EIGHT Basic Physiological Needs
36 Activity and Exercise, **168**
37 Quality and Patient Safety, **174**
38 Hygiene, **179**
39 Cardiopulmonary Functioning and Oxygenation, **188**
40 Fluid, Electrolyte, and Acid–Base Balances, **201**
41 Sleep, **212**
42 Nutrition, **220**
43 Urinary Elimination, **231**
44 Bowel Elimination, **241**

UNIT NINE Patients with Special Needs
45 Mobility and Immobility, **251**
46 Skin Integrity and Wound Care, **257**
47 Sensory Alterations, **265**
48 Care of Surgical Patients, **271**

Copyright © 2019 Elsevier Canada, a division of Reed Elsevier Canada, Ltd.

Introduction

The *Study Guide to accompany Canadian Fundamentals of Nursing*, Sixth Edition, has been developed to encourage independent learning for beginning nursing students. As you begin to read the text, you may note a difference in style and format from other books you've used in the past. The terms are new, and the focus of the content is different. You may be wondering, "How will I possibly learn all of the material in this chapter?" The essential objective of this study guide is to assist you in this endeavour—to help you learn what you need to know and then self-test with hundreds of review questions.

This study guide follows the text chapter for chapter. Whatever chapter your instructor assigns, you will use the same chapter number in this study guide. The outline format was designed to help you learn to read nursing content more effectively and with greater understanding. Each chapter of this study guide has the following sections to assist you to comprehend and recall.

The *Preliminary Reading* section is designed to teach prereading strategies. You need to become familiar with the chapter by first reading the chapter title, the key concepts and key terms, and all headings, as well as review all photographs, drawings, tables, and boxes. This can be done rather quickly and will give you an overall idea of the content of the chapter.

The *Comprehensive Understanding* section is next and is in outline format. This will prove to be a very valuable tool, not only as you first read the chapter but also as you review for tests. This outline identifies the topics and main ideas of each chapter as an aid to concentration, comprehension, and retaining textbook information. By completing this outline, you will learn to "pull out" key information in the chapter. As you write the answers in the study guide, you will be reinforcing that content. Once completed, this outline will serve as a review tool for exams. After you have completed this section, you can check the answers on the Evolve website.

The *Review Questions* in each chapter provide a valuable means of testing and reinforcing your knowledge of the material read and the answers written in the outline. Each question is multiple choice. As a further aid for independent learning, each answer requires a rationale (the reason why the option you selected is correct). After you have completed the review questions, you can check the answers on the Evolve website.

Chapters 26, 27, 29, 31, and 36 to 48 include exercises based on the care plans found in the text. These exercises provide practice in synthesizing the nursing process and critical thinking as you, the nurse, care for patients. Taking one aspect of the nursing process, you will be asked to imagine you are the nurse in the case study and to think about what knowledge, experiences, standards, and attitudes might be used in caring for the patient. Write your answers in the appropriate boxes and check them against the answer key.

When you finish answering the review questions and synthesis exercises, take a few minutes for self-evaluation. If you answered a question incorrectly, begin to analyze the thoughts that led you to the wrong answer:

- Did you miss the key word or phrase?
- Did you read into something that wasn't stated?
- Did you not understand the subject matter?
- Did you use an incorrect rationale for selecting your response?

Each incorrect response is an opportunity to learn. Go back to the text and reread any content that is still unclear. In the long run, it will be a time-saving activity.

The learning activities presented in this study guide will assist you in completing the semester with a firm understanding of nursing concepts and processes that you can rely on for all of your professional career.

Copyright © 2019 Elsevier Canada, a division of Reed Elsevier Canada, Ltd.

1 Health and Wellness

PRELIMINARY READING

Chapter 1, pages 1–17

COMPREHENSIVE UNDERSTANDING

Conceptualizations of Health

Classifications of health conceptualizations

1. List five different conceptualizations of health.
   a. ______
   b. ______
   c. ______
   d. ______
   e. ______

Historical Approaches to Health in Canada

2. Historically, the three different approaches to health in Canada have been *medical*, *behavioural*, and *socio-environmental*. Identify the distinguishing features of each of these approaches.
   a. Medical:
   b. Behavioural:
   c. Socioenvironmental:

3. Identify the contributions of the following Canadian documents to the understanding of health and health determinants.
   a. *Lalonde Report*:
   b. *Ottawa Charter*:
   c. *Epp Report*:
   d. *Strategies for Population Health*:
   e. *Toronto Charter*:
   f. *Bangkok Charter*:
   g. *Jakarta Declaration*:

Determinants of Health and Social Determinants of Health

4. Identify 12 major *determinants of health*, as outlined by Health Canada, the *Ottawa Charter*, and the *Toronto Charter*.

Copyright © 2019 Elsevier Canada, a division of Reed Elsevier Canada, Ltd.

Strategies to Influence Health Determinants

5. The concepts of *health promotion* and *disease prevention* are distinct yet interrelated. Briefly explain each one.

   a. Health promotion:

   ____

   ____

   b. Disease prevention:

   ____

   ____

6. Define the three levels of prevention, and give an example of each.

   a. Primary prevention:

   ____

   ____

   b. Secondary prevention:

   ____

   ____

   c. Tertiary prevention:

   ____

   ____

Health Promotion Strategies

7. Define the five health promotion strategies contained in the *Ottawa Charter*, and give examples of activities in each strategy.

   a. Build healthy public policy:

   ____

   ____

   b. Create supportive environments:

   ____

   ____

   c. Strengthen community action:

   ____

   ____

   d. Develop personal skills:

   ____

   ____

   e. Reorient health services:

   ____

   ____

Population Health Promotion Model: Putting It All Together

8. What are the four major elements of the Population Health Promotion Model?

   a. ______________________________

   b. ______________________________

   c. ______________________________

   d. ______________________________

9. Provide an example of how you might use this model in your practice.

   ____

   ____

   ____

REVIEW QUESTIONS

Select the appropriate answer, and cite the rationale for choosing that particular answer.

1. Which of the following was the influential document that marked the shift from a lifestyle to a socioenvironmental approach to health?
   a. *Lalonde Report*
   b. *Jakarta Declaration*
   c. *Toronto Charter*
   d. *Ottawa Charter*

Answer: ______________ Rationale: ______________

____

____

2. Which of the following major determinants of health would be consistent with a socioenvironmental view of health? *(Select all that apply.)*
   a. Income and social status
   b. Employment and working conditions
   c. Physiologic predisposition to disease
   d. Self-imposed behavioural risk factors

Answer: ______________ Rationale: ______________

____

____

3. Which of the following is an example of intersectoral collaboration?
   a. Clients, municipal authorities, and social services develop strategies and policies to address housing challenges for persons with addictions.
   b. A patient and a physician jointly decide on the best treatment plan to address the patient's health concerns.

Copyright © 2019 Elsevier Canada, a division of Reed Elsevier Canada, Ltd.

c. Physicians and nurses engage in joint patient care rounds to discuss patients.
d. Persons with multiple sclerosis form a local chapter to support families and patients and liaise with the national organization.

Answer:______________Rationale:______________

4. Healthy Babies programs that provide mothers with information and support to avoid injuries and obesity in babies are an example of which of the following?
   a. Health promotion
   b. Primary prevention
   c. Secondary prevention
   d. Tertiary prevention

Answer:______________Rationale:______________

5. Which of the following statements does *not* accurately characterize health promotion?
   a. Health promotion reorients health care services.
   b. The primary emphasis of health promotion is on assisting the individual to develop healthy behaviours.
   c. Health promotion strategies utilize research and education related to development of programming for health.
   d. Health promotion positions health within a sociopolitical context that considers what is needed to strengthen public and individual capabilities for health.

Answer:______________Rationale:______________

6. Which of the following is a key concept in the medical model?
   a. Stability
   b. Empowerment
   c. Justice
   d. Prevention

Answer:______________Rationale:______________

7. Which of the following prerequisites for health has also been included as a metaparadigm concept in nursing?
   a. Sustainable environments
   b. Stable ecosystem
   c. Social justice
   d. Food and income

Answer:______________Rationale:______________

8. Which of the following exemplifies empowerment?
   a. A nurse provides a patient with instructions regarding postconcussion follow-up.
   b. Persons who have been homeless provide oversight of the management of a housing cooperative for others who are homeless.
   c. Community workers in an impoverished neighborhood organize events based on prior research.
   d. Health workers in an Indigenous community provide services and services access identical to those elsewhere in Canada.

Answer:______________Rationale:______________

9. A medical approach to health is to health services as a behavioural approach is to which of the following?
   a. Income and social status
   b. Employment and working conditions
   c. Physical environments
   d. Personal health practices

Answer:______________Rationale:______________

10. Understanding the context in which health behaviours occur most accurately reflects which approach to health?
   a. Behavioural
   b. Medical
   c. Socioenvironmental
   d. Primary prevention

Answer:______________Rationale:______________

Copyright © 2019 Elsevier Canada, a division of Reed Elsevier Canada, Ltd.

2 The Canadian Health Care Delivery System

PRELIMINARY READING

Chapter 2, pages 18–33

COMPREHENSIVE UNDERSTANDING

Evolution of the Canadian Health Care System

1. Canada has constructed a social safety net for the protection of its citizens. Medicare is an important part of this safety net. Briefly explain the role of the following in the development of Medicare.

   a. *British North America Act:*

   b. Great Depression:

   c. Tommy Douglas:

   d. *Medical Care Act* (1966):

   e. *Canada Health Act* (1984):

2. What are the original five principles enshrined in the *Canada Health Act*?

3. Identify four calls to action that were directed at health in the Truth and Reconciliation Commission of Canada report?

The Organization and Governance of Health Care

4. Under the *Canadian Constitution Act*, administration and delivery of health care services are primarily provincial or territorial responsibilities. The federal government, however, continues to have a role. Briefly explain the following:

   a. The four areas of federal jurisdiction for health care in Canada:

   b. The role of the provincial and territorial governments in the organization and delivery of health care:

Trends and Reforms in Canada's Health Care System

5. Recently, some provinces have moved toward *recentralization* of health care. To what does recentralization refer?

6. For 2017–2018, a new federal funding model was introduced that bases payment upon __________.

Right to Health Care

7. What four working conditions can Canadian health care workers reasonably expect?

Copyright © 2019 Elsevier Canada, a division of Reed Elsevier Canada, Ltd.

Primary Health Care

8. Explain the difference between *primary care* (PC) and *primary health care* (PHC).

9. List the four pillars of PHC.
   a.
   b.
   c.
   d.

10. Describe three types of barriers that are challenges to IPC in primary health care.

Settings for Health Care Delivery

11. Explain the role of each of the following institutions in delivering health care.
    a. Hospitals:
    b. Long-term care facilities:
    c. Psychiatric facilities:
    d. Rehabilitation centres:

12. Explain the role of each of the following in delivering health care in the community.
    a. Public health:
    b. Physician offices:
    c. Community health centres and clinics:
    d. Assisted living:
    e. Home care:
    f. Adult day support programs:
    g. Community and voluntary agencies:
    h. Occupational health:
    i. Hospice and palliative care:
    j. Parish nursing:

Levels of Care

13. List and briefly describe the five levels of health care.
    a.
    b.
    c.
    d.
    e.

Copyright © 2019 Elsevier Canada, a division of Reed Elsevier Canada, Ltd.

14. Explain *primary care*, *secondary care*, and *tertiary care*.

____

____

____

____

____

____

Challenges to the Health Care System

15. Describe three cost accelerators in the Canadian health care system.

    a. ______________________________________

    ____

    b. ______________________________________

    ____

    c. ______________________________________

    ____

REVIEW QUESTIONS

Select the appropriate answer, and cite the rationale for choosing that particular answer.

1. When the *Canada Health Act* of 1984 amalgamated the previous acts of 1957 and 1966, it added which principle to the existing four?
   a. Accessibility
   b. Comprehensiveness
   c. Portability
   d. Public administration

Answer: ____________ Rationale: ____________

____

____

2. The amount of money (public and private) Canada spent on health care per capita in 2016 was approximately how much?
   a. $3839
   b. $4548
   c. $5614
   d. $6299

Answer: ____________ Rationale: ____________

____

____

3. A 16-year-old student sees a physician at a walk-in clinic to find out if she is pregnant. This service can be best described as an example of which of the following?
   a. Primary care
   b. Primary health care
   c. Tertiary care
   d. Secondary care

Answer: ____________ Rationale: ____________

____

____

4. The 16-year-old student attends a community program on prenatal health for teenage mothers. The program is taught by a nurse, a nutritionist, and a social worker. This service can best be described as an example of which of the following?
   a. Primary care
   b. Primary health care
   c. Tertiary care
   d. Secondary care

Answer: ____________ Rationale: ____________

____

____

5. Which of the following is true? *(Select all that apply.)*
   a. Most nurses work in institutional settings in Canada.
   b. Most RN nursing graduates are degree prepared.
   c. More RNs work in community than in long-term care.
   d. The ratio of nurses in Canada is one RN for every 119 persons.

Answer: ____________ Rationale: ____________

____

____

Copyright © 2019 Elsevier Canada, a division of Reed Elsevier Canada, Ltd.

3 The Development of Nursing in Canada

PRELIMINARY READING

Chapter 3, pages 34–47

COMPREHENSIVE UNDERSTANDING

Why Nursing History Matters

1. Identify five reasons why nursing history is important.

Care of Strangers: The Early History of Nursing

2. What was the contribution of Mme. Hébert to health care in the new colony?

3. Describe the contributions of Jeanne Mance to health care and the early development of Canada.

4. Describe the beginnings and mission of the Grey Nuns.

Health care in the west and the Grey Nuns

5. The Grey Nuns travelled from Montreal and cared for the sick in which parts of Canada?

   a. ______

   b. ______

   c. ______

   d. ______

6. Describe the main themes in Florence Nightingale's *Notes on Nursing.*

Globalization and the Emergence of Modern Nursing

7. Discuss the sociopolitical developments that allowed Canadian missionary nurses into China in the 1880s.

8. Describe the roles and areas of expertise that nurses in remote areas of Canada developed.

9. Since the 1960s and 1970s, the nursing profession has become increasingly aware of the need for ______ ______, and ______ ______ in nursing.

Nursing Education in Canada

10. What was the main reason for establishing the first Canadian nursing schools?

11. Describe the growth of hospital nursing schools in the late nineteenth century.

12. What were the goals of the founders of the ICN?

    a. ______

    b. ______

    c. ______

13. The Canadian Nurses Association (CNA) became a federation of provincial associations in which year?
    a. 1924
    b. 1907
    c. 1930
    d. 1899

Copyright © 2019 Elsevier Canada, a division of Reed Elsevier Canada, Ltd.

14. For almost a century, the ICN has sustained its place as the key organization for

____

______________________________.

15. Licensure laws are designed to protect the public against unqualified and incompetent practitioners. Highlight the differences between permissive and mandatory legislation.

____

____

____

16. What two values underpinned the first CNA Code of Ethics for nurses?

____

____

17. How did the struggle for women's rights influence nursing?

____

____

____

18. When and where was the first university undergraduate nursing program in Canada established?

____

____

____

Health Care and Educational Reform

19. Describe the following reports.

   a. *Weir Report*:

   ____

   ____

   b. The report of the Royal Commission on Health Services of 1964:

   ____

   ____

   c. *Spotlight on Nursing Education*:

   ____

   ____

20. Describe the major events in the movement toward *baccalaureate as entry-to-practice*.

____

____

____

____

Influence of Periods of Social Upheaval on Nursing

21. In the first quarter of the twentieth century, women in western Canada became seriously involved in commenting on needs in health and education, and developed organizations to put forward their ideas. What five Albertan women petitioned the Supreme Court of Canada for women's rights?

   a. ______________________________

   b. ______________________________

   c. ______________________________

   d. ______________________________

   e. ______________________________

22. Describe the relationship between the Canadian Red Cross and university programs in nursing.

____

____

____

23. The Great Depression brought ______________ and ______________ to nurses.

24. How did World War II affect health education?

____

____

____

25. Describe the development of graduate programs during the years following World War II.

____

____

____

Nursing education today

26. Where does the responsibility for monitoring standards of nursing education lie?

____

____

27. A master's degree in nursing is necessary for

____

______________________________.

28. Describe the focus of nurse practitioners (NPs).

____

____

29. Nurses with doctorates can ______________________________

______________________________.

Copyright © 2019 Elsevier Canada, a division of Reed Elsevier Canada, Ltd.

Conclusion

30. Describe the fundamental principle of early French-Canadian hospitals that is strongly advocated by Canadian nurses today.

____

____

REVIEW QUESTIONS

Select the appropriate answer, and cite the rationale for choosing that particular answer.

1. Which of the following statements accurately describes mandatory legislation for nurses?
   a. Defines scope of practice and protects the title of registered nurse
   b. Applies only to registered nurses (RNs)
   c. Offers nurses a choice as to whether they need to be licensed in their jurisdiction
   d. Applies only to nurses in advanced practice or those with graduate degrees

Answer:______________ Rationale:______________

____

____

2. The first visiting nurses in Canada were _____.
   a. led by Jeanne Mance in 1642
   b. the first three Augustinian nuns in 1639
   c. Marie Rollet Hébert and her surgeon-apothecary husband in 1617
   d. the Grey Nuns under Marguerite d'Youville in 1737

Answer:______________ Rationale:______________

____

____

3. Which of the following is *not* attributed to Florence Nightingale?
   a. Dramatically reduced morbidity and mortality rates among the wounded
   b. Advocated baccalaureate level university education for nurses
   c. Introduced nursing to the British army during the Crimean War
   d. Made nursing an acceptable field of work for middle- and upper-class women outside the home

Answer:______________ Rationale:______________

____

____

4. The first undergraduate degree program in nursing in Canada was developed where?
   a. St. Francis Xavier University
   b. University of Toronto
   c. University of Alberta
   d. University of British Columbia

Answer:______________ Rationale:______________

____

____

5. Which struggle helped nurses secure laws to regulate their profession in Canada?
   a. Public health
   b. Crimean War
   c. Women's rights
   d. University education

Answer:______________ Rationale:______________

____

____

Copyright © 2019 Elsevier Canada, a division of Reed Elsevier Canada, Ltd.

4 Community Health Nursing Practice

PRELIMINARY READING

Chapter 4, pages 48–62

COMPREHENSIVE UNDERSTANDING

1. Community health nursing care focuses on ______________________________.

Promoting the Health of Populations and Community Groups

2. Distinguish between a *population* and a *community*, and give an example of each.

3. Compare the characteristics of a *healthy population* and a *healthy community.*

Community Health Nursing Practice

4. Describe the scope of *community health nursing practice.*

5. Define *social justice.*

6. Briefly explain the nursing focus in *primary health care* (PHC).

7. Briefly explain the nursing focus on *empowerment* in community health nursing as guided by PHC.

8. What health challenges would outpost nurses most likely encounter in the community?

9. Briefly describe the contributions of public health and population health to *public health nursing.*

10. A strong theoretical foundation for *home health nursing* is provided by ______________________________.

11. Briefly describe key distinctions between *public health nursing* and *home health nursing.*

    a. Public health nursing:

    b. Home health nursing:

The Changing Focus of Community Health Nursing Practice

Vulnerable populations

12. *Vulnerable populations* of patients are those who are ______________________________.

Copyright © 2019 Elsevier Canada, a division of Reed Elsevier Canada, Ltd.

13. Explain how a nurse approaches diversity to provide culturally sensitive, competent, and safe care.

14. List some of the reasons why vulnerable populations typically experience poorer health outcomes.

15. Briefly describe the following vulnerable groups, and identify the circumstances that contribute to their vulnerability.

    a. Poor and homeless people:

    b. People in precarious circumstances:

    c. People with chronic conditions and disabilities:

    d. People who engage in stigmatizing risk behaviours:

Standards, competencies, roles, and activities in community health nursing

16. A nurse in a community health practice must have a variety of skills and knowledge to assist individuals and families within the community, as well as communities broadly. Briefly explain the competencies the community nurse needs to develop.

    a. Communication:

    b. Facilitation:

    c. Leadership:

    d. Advocacy:

    e. Consultation:

    f. Team building and collaboration:

    g. Building capacity:

    h. Building coalitions and networks:

    i. Outreach:

    j. Resource management, planning, coordination:

    k. Case management:

    l. Care/counselling:

    m. Referral and follow-up:

    n. Screening:

    o. Surveillance:

Copyright © 2019 Elsevier Canada, a division of Reed Elsevier Canada, Ltd.

p. Health threat response:

q. Health education:

r. Community development:

s. Policy development and implementation:

t. Research and evaluation:

Community Assessment

17. The community is viewed as having three components. Briefly explain each one.

a. Locale or structure:

b. Social systems:

c. People:

18. Briefly describe each of the following strategies to assess the locale or structure of a community and the kind of data that you would expect to obtain when using each strategy.

a. Windshield or walking survey:

b. Key informant interviews:

c. Population data review:

Promoting Patients' Health

19. The challenge is how to promote and protect the patient's health, whether within the context of the community or with the community as the focus. The most important theme to consider, to be an effective community health nurse, is to ______________

______________.

REVIEW QUESTIONS

Select the appropriate answer, and cite the rationale for choosing that particular answer.

1. Which of the following would *not* typically be considered an example of PHC? *(Select all that apply.)*
   a. Lunchtime nutrition and activity program in an inner-city school run by nurses, nutritionists, social workers, and teachers
   b. A rehabilitation program in a hospital provided by physiotherapists, physicians, nurses, and social workers for patients and families recovering from a stroke
   c. Activities provided by child care workers in a day care centre at a corporation
   d. A well-baby clinic conducted by nurses and nutritionists for new mothers at a neighbourhood health centre
   e. Clinic with physicians, nurses, chiropractors, and physiotherapists that specializes in treating back pain

Answer: ______________ Rationale: ______________

2. Among the communication skills needed to provide nursing care to community patients is the ability to do which of the following?
   a. Clarify patient values and care expectations
   b. Follow medical prescriptions in many settings
   c. Manage generational interfamilial conflict
   d. Speak the patient's language or dialects

Answer: ______________ Rationale: ______________

3. What is specific to people who are poor and homeless?
   a. They have a high incidence of mental illness and substance abuse
   b. They have more resources than low-income people
   c. They eat nutritious food
   d. They have great trust in health and social services

Answer: ______________ Rationale: ______________

Copyright © 2019 Elsevier Canada, a division of Reed Elsevier Canada, Ltd.

4. When the community health nurse refers patients to appropriate resources, and monitors and coordinates the extent and adequacy of services to meet family health care needs, the nurse is functioning in which role?
   a. Collaborator
   b. Educator
   c. Consultant
   d. Coordinator

Answer: ______________ Rationale: ______________

____

____

5. Which of the following is *not* identified as a challenge in community health nursing?
   a. Increased task orientation, specialization, and working in silos
   b. Staying current on health information
   c. Limited demand for acute care in the community
   d. Conflict between prescribed programs and community partnership activities

Answer: ______________ Rationale: ______________

____

____

Copyright © 2019 Elsevier Canada, a division of Reed Elsevier Canada, Ltd.

5 Theoretical Foundations of Nursing Practice

PRELIMINARY READING

Chapter 5, pages 63–74

COMPREHENSIVE UNDERSTANDING

1. Define the terms *theory* and *nursing theory*, and explain why knowledge of nursing theory can help nurses become better practitioners.

Early Nursing Practice and the Emergence of Theory

2. Briefly describe how developments in science and technology affected the development of nursing as a science.

3. Explain the relationship between the development of nursing theory and the development of curriculum for nursing education.

Nursing Process

4. Describe the four basic steps of the *nursing process.*

   a. Assessment:

   b. Planning:

   c. Intervention:

   d. Evaluation:

5. The relationship between clinical judgement and nursing process is ____________.

Conceptual Frameworks

6. Briefly describe how systematic thinking using conceptual nursing models differs from linear reasoning processes.

Metaparadigm Concepts

7. Explain the importance of each *metaparadigm concept* for the clinical reasoning process in nursing.

   a. Client and person:

   b. Environment:

   c. Health:

   d. Nursing:

Copyright © 2019 Elsevier Canada, a division of Reed Elsevier Canada, Ltd.

8. For each metaparadigm concept, identify at least two possible ways it might be defined for the purpose of guiding nursing practice.

   a. Client and person:

   ____

   ____

   b. Environment:

   ____

   ____

   c. Health:

   ____

   ____

   d. Nursing:

   ____

   ____

Philosophy of Nursing Science

9. Thomas S. Kuhn's ideas about *paradigms* helped nurses understand the scientific basis of nursing not simply as theoretical propositions but as

   ____

   ______________________________.

10. *Chaos theory* provided nurses with a new way to think about

    ______________________________.

Ways of Knowing in Nursing Practice

11. List four forms of knowledge identified by Carper that have contributed to excellent nursing practice.

    a. ______________________________

    b. ______________________________

    c. ______________________________

    d. ______________________________

Paradigm Debates Within Nursing

12. The two distinct paradigms that have been associated with debates surrounding nursing's theoretical development are ______________ and ______________

    ______________________________.

Nursing Diagnosis

13. Identify advantages and disadvantages of adopting a fixed list of diagnostic categories for nursing care.

    a. Advantages:

    ____

    ____

    ____

    b. Disadvantages:

    ____

    ____

    ____

Reflections on Conceptualizing Nursing

Instead of arguing the advantages of one nursing theory over another, nursing scholars of today appreciate the creativity of their predecessors within the constrained conceptual contexts in which they were expected to operate.

Major Theoretical Models

14. Identify one characteristic of each of the following categories of theoretical models.

    a. Practice-based theories:

    ____

    ____

    b. Needs theories:

    ____

    ____

    c. Interactionist theories:

    ____

    ____

    d. Systems theories:

    ____

    ____

    e. Simultaneity theories:

    ____

    ____

15. Name one theory or theorist as an example for each of the categories listed in question 14.

    a. ______________________________

    b. ______________________________

    c. ______________________________

    d. ______________________________

    e. ______________________________

16. *Praxis* is a dialogue representing the dynamic interaction between theorizing and clinical practice. This newer form of theorizing does not seek ______________ truths about nursing practice because ______________________________.

Copyright © 2019 Elsevier Canada, a division of Reed Elsevier Canada, Ltd.

REVIEW QUESTIONS

Select the appropriate answer, and cite the rationale for choosing that particular answer.

1. Which of the following is *not* an intended outcome of a grand theory?
   a. To provide guidance for specific nursing interventions
   b. To provide a framework for broad ideas about nursing
   c. To provide a structural framework within which smaller range theories can be developed
   d. To stimulate critical thinking about nursing ideas

Answer:______________ Rationale:______________

2. Which of the following is *not* an intended outcome of a prescriptive theory? *(Select all that apply.)*
   a. To provide insight into general and broad phenomena
   b. To be action oriented
   c. To test validity
   d. To describe and explain a phenomenon
   e. To predict the consequence of a specific intervention

Answer:______________ Rationale:______________

3. Which nursing theorist's model conceptualizes the person as an adaptive system?
   a. Virginia Henderson
   b. Rosemary Parse
   c. Hildegard Peplau
   d. Sister Callista Roy

Answer:______________ Rationale:______________

4. Which nursing theorist's model conceptualizes the person as an irreducible energy field, coextensive with the universe?
   a. Adam's interactionist theory
   b. Orem's self-care theory
   c. Rogers's simultaneity theory
   d. Watson's transpersonal theory

Answer:______________ Rationale:______________

5. Which of the following levels of abstraction is *not* part of Liaschenko's ideas about nursing knowledge?
   a. Knowing the case
   b. Knowing the patient
   c. Knowing the disease
   d. Knowing the person

Answer:______________ Rationale:______________

Copyright © 2019 Elsevier Canada, a division of Reed Elsevier Canada, Ltd.

6 Evidence-Informed Practice

PRELIMINARY READING

Chapter 6, pages 75–86

COMPREHENSIVE UNDERSTANDING

Why Evidence?

1. Compare *evidence-based decision making* with *evidence-informed practice.*

____

2. What is the purpose of evidence-informed decision making?

____

Relationship Between Evidence-Informed Decision Making, Research, and Quality Improvement (QI)

3. Explain the differences between *evidence-informed decision making* and *quality improvement.*

____

Development of Nursing Knowledge

4. In applying evidence to practice, it is critical that nurses have the ability to _______________.

Researching the Evidence

5. Describe a PICO question.

____

Collect the best evidence

6. Describe where and how to find research studies in nursing.

____

Research literacy: critique the evidence

7. How is research evidence assessed for applicability in practice?

____

8. The typical research article has the following parts. Briefly explain each section.

   a. Introduction: _______________

   b. Methods: _______________

   c. Results or conclusions: _______________

   d. Clinical implications: _______________

Integrate the evidence

9. Using an evidence-informed practice approach helps you improve _______________.

Evaluate the Practice Decision or Change

10. What two questions must be asked to evaluate the effect of an intervention?

   a. _______________

   b. _______________

Support for Evidence-Informed Practice

11. Identify two reasons for the importance of evidence-informed practice.

____

Copyright © 2019 Elsevier Canada, a division of Reed Elsevier Canada, Ltd.

The Development of Research in Nursing

12. Nursing research involves ______________________________

______________________________.

Its purpose is to ______________________________.

13. Briefly describe the relationship between *research* and *theory*.

____

____

____

The History of Nursing Research in Canada

14. Briefly explain the significance of each of the following:

a. The work of Florence Nightingale:

____

____

____

b. The development of master's and doctoral degree programs in nursing:

____

____

____

15. To what does *Tri-Council* refer?

____

____

Nursing Research

16. The research process must start with a ______________

______________________________.

Research Designs

17. The two broad approaches to research are ______________

and ______________________________.

Quantitative nursing research

18. Briefly describe the three requirements of a *true experiment.*

____

____

____

19. A *quasi experiment* is one in which groups are formed and the conditions are controlled, but

____

____

______________________________.

20. Surveys are designed to

____

______________________________.

Qualitative nursing research

21. Explain how the applicability of the findings of a qualitative study to a similar situation (transferability) is assessed.

____

____

____

Conducting nursing research

22. Who should conduct clinical nursing research?

____

____

Ethical Issues in Research

23. Describe the purpose and responsibilities of a research ethics board.

____

____

____

24. What does *informed consent* mean in relation to research participants?

____

____

25. Briefly describe the five guiding ethical principles for research in Canada.

a. ______________________________

b. ______________________________

c. ______________________________

d. ______________________________

e. ______________________________

Applying Research Findings to Nursing Practice

26. What does evidence-informed practice de-emphasize?

____

____

____

Copyright © 2019 Elsevier Canada, a division of Reed Elsevier Canada, Ltd.

REVIEW QUESTIONS

Select the appropriate answer, and cite the rationale for choosing that particular answer.

1. The researcher's refusal to disclose the names of subjects is termed which of the following?
   a. Respect for privacy and confidentiality
   b. Minimizing harm
   c. Informed consent
   d. Balancing harms and benefits

Answer:_______________ Rationale:_______________

2. What is the purpose of a research ethics board?
   a. Ensure that federal funds are equitably appropriated
   b. Conduct research benefiting the public
   c. Determine the risk status of patients in research projects
   d. Ensure that ethical principles are being upheld

Answer:_______________ Rationale:_______________

3. Which of the following would be described as research? (*Select all that apply.*)
   a. Systematic study of the response of patients to different approaches to pain control
   b. Chart audit by nursing staff to determine frequency of inappropriate medication administration
   c. Staff review of existing studies and best practices to find the best methods for wound care in the clinical setting
   d. Exploration of what persons over 65 years of age view as "good health"
   e. Reading the abstract of the report

Answer:_______________ Rationale:_______________

4. Which statement concerning research articles is accurate?
   a. Nursing textbooks are current sources of information.
   b. Systematic reviews and meta-analysis of randomized controlled trials (RCTs) provide the best evidence.
   c. RCTs do not provide scientific evidence.
   d. Peer-reviewed articles have been reviewed by a panel of nurses before publication.

Answer:_______________ Rationale:_______________

5. Which of the following does a research article *not* include?
   a. A summary of literature used to identify the research problem
   b. The researcher's interpretation of the study results
   c. A summary of other research studies with the same results
   d. A description of methods used to conduct the study

Answer:_______________ Rationale:_______________

Copyright © 2019 Elsevier Canada, a division of Reed Elsevier Canada, Ltd.

7 Nursing Values and Ethics

PRELIMINARY READING

Chapter 7, pages 87–100

COMPREHENSIVE UNDERSTANDING

1. A *value* is a

____

____.

2. *Ethics* is the study of

____

____.

Values

3. *Moral development* is a process throughout childhood and adolescence when people learn to

____

____.

4. *Value conflict* occurs when

____

____.

5. *Values clarification* is

____

____.

6. Identify three values clarification questions.

a. ____

b. ____

c. ____

Ethics

7. Define *ethics* or *morality.*

____

____

____

____

8. A *code of ethics* serves

____

____.

9. Identify and briefly describe the seven values that must be upheld by Canadian nurses according to the Canadian Nurses Association.

a. ____

____

b. ____

____

c. ____

____

d. ____

____

e. ____

____

f. ____

____

g. ____

____

10. Define the following terms, and explain how they apply to the role of the nurse.

a. *Responsibility*:

____

____

b. *Accountability*:

____

____

c. *Advocacy*:

____

____

Copyright © 2019 Elsevier Canada, a division of Reed Elsevier Canada, Ltd.

Ethical theory

11. Define the following terms.
   a. *Deontology*:
   b. *Utilitarianism*:
   c. *Bioethics*:
   d. *Autonomy*:
   e. *Beneficence*:
   f. *Nonmaleficence*:
   g. *Justice*:
   h. *Social justice*:
   i. *Feminist ethics*:
   j. *Relational ethics*:
   k. *Environment*:
   l. *Embodiment*:
   m. *Mutuality*:
   n. *Engagement*:

Ethical Analysis and Nursing

12. An *ethical dilemma* is

13. Briefly describe each of the seven steps in the processing of an ethical dilemma.
   a. Step 1:
   b. Step 2:
   c. Step 3:
   d. Step 4:
   e. Step 5:
   f. Step 6:
   g. Step 7:

Copyright © 2019 Elsevier Canada, a division of Reed Elsevier Canada, Ltd.

Ethical Issues in Nursing Practice

14. Explain the following patient care issues and how they apply to nursing.

    a. *Medical futility*:

    ____

    ____

    b. *Advance care planning (ACP)*:

    ____

    ____

    c. *Medical assistance in dying (MAID)*:

    ____

    ____

15. When using social media, it is important to remember that it is not ____________ but resides within the ______________________________.

REVIEW QUESTIONS

Select the appropriate answer, and cite the rationale for choosing that particular answer.

1. Nursing codes of ethics fulfill which of the following purposes?
   a. They help nurses and the public understand professional nursing conduct.
   b. They outline actions to be implemented in specific nursing care situations.
   c. They define the scope of nursing practice on a national level.
   d. They define the roles of the nurse, the patient, other health care providers, and society.

Answer: ____________ Rationale: ____________

____

____

2. Identify which of the following statements are *not* accurate regarding advance care planning. *(Select all that apply.)*
   a. Advance care planning offers direction in care goals to health care providers.
   b. Advance care planning involves two persons: the patient and the physician.
   c. Advance care planning can identify others who can make decisions on behalf of the patient.
   d. Another term for advance care planning is *physician-assisted dying*.

Answer: ____________ Rationale: ____________

____

____

3. A family is faced with many decisions regarding their seriously ill and very premature infant. They are informed of the medical risks and benefits of treatment, including the futility of further aggressive intervention. Despite this information, the family struggles emotionally with the decision to discontinue further aggressive intervention and asks for more time to make their decision. The nurse brings this request to the attention of the team and advocates for the family. Which theme in relational ethics is the nurse exemplifying through this action?
   a. Environment
   b. Autonomy
   c. Embodiment
   d. Justice

Answer: ____________ Rationale: ____________

____

____

4. You are working with the parents of a seriously ill newborn. Surgery has been proposed for the infant, but the chances of success are unclear. In helping the parents resolve this ethical conflict, you know that the next step is which of the following?
   a. Exploring reasonable courses of action
   b. Collecting all available information about the situation
   c. Clarifying values related to the cause of the dilemma
   d. Identifying people who can solve the difficulty

Answer: ____________ Rationale: ____________

____

____

5. The goal of informed consent is to protect the patient's right to which of the following?
   a. Autonomy
   b. Beneficence
   c. Ethic of care
   d. Advocacy

Answer: ____________ Rationale: ____________

____

____

Copyright © 2019 Elsevier Canada, a division of Reed Elsevier Canada, Ltd.

8 Legal Implications in Nursing Practice

PRELIMINARY READING

Chapter 8, pages 101–114

COMPREHENSIVE UNDERSTANDING

Legal Limits of Nursing

1. The legal guidelines that nurses must follow are derived from the following. Briefly explain each one.

   a. *Statute law*:
   Created by elective legislation bodies such as parliment, provincial, territorial, legislatures

   b. *Nursing practice acts*:
   health professional acts from prov. & terr legislative that defines scope of nursing practices by sett edu req by distinguishing between med & nursing pract & provide def of nursing

   c. *Standards of care*:
   legal guidelines for nursing practice; provide safe & appropriate patient care

   d. *Common law*:
   A system that deals with private law issues (criminal law)

2. *Standards of care* are the legal guidelines for nursing practice and are defined by the
   expectation of nursing to provide safe & appropriate patient care. If not nurses can face legal action. Statue & laws of broad application apply to human rights, privacy & confidential negligence

3. *Nursing practice acts* establish
   that all nurses know & follow from the regulatory bodies & prov & terr define nursing practice specifically scope of nurs practice, edu

4. In a negligence lawsuit, standards of care are used to determine
   whether the nurse has acted as any reasonably prudent nurse in a similar setting w/ same credentials would act

Legal Liability Issues in Nursing Practice

5. Define *tort*.
   cival wrong committed against a person or property

6. Define the following:

   a. *Assault*: - no contact necessary
   conduct (physical/verbal) that creates in another person apprehensive or fear of iniminent harmful & offensive contact

   b. *Battery*:
   intentional physical contact w/ a person w/out that persons consent

   c. *Invasion of privacy*:
   protects the patients right to be free from unwanted intrusion into his/her private affairs

   d. *False imprisonment*:
   protects persons individual liberty & basic rights. ex putting up the guard rails on bed

7. Describe three precautions that must be taken to protect confidentiality of patient information when using computers, portable devices, and social media.
   - cards & passwords not shared
   - dont post related to work
   - maintain prof bounderies & not connect on media

8. Define *negligence*.
   conduct that doesnt meet standard of care established

9. Briefly explain how a nurse can avoid being liable for negligence.
   proper med practise, notify & communicate w/ other staff, know & follow rules, unsure; ask, shred documents, confident care, proper orientation, document properly

10. Describe the difference between the *tort of negligence* and *criminal negligence charges*.
    nurse showed inadvertence, thoughtlessness or inattention where they didnt carry out their duty/care to patient & the patient is harmed/injurred. Criminal → reckless disregard for lives & safety of another person (assult, manslaughter, death)

Copyright © 2019 Elsevier Canada, a division of Reed Elsevier Canada, Ltd.

11. The following factors must be verified for consent to be legally valid.
    a. patient must have legal & mental capacity
    b. consent given voluntary w/out
    c. patient must understand the risks/benefits of produre/treatment
12. *Informed consent* is a person's agreement to allow med action to happen based on a full disclosure of the likely risks & benefits, & understanding consequences of refusal
13. The following factors provide adequate information for the patient to formulate a decision and are required to have met the standard of informed consent.
    a. brief/complete explanation of procedure/treatment ~~assiting w/ procedure~~
    b. names/qualifications of ppl peforming & assisting w/procedure
    c. description of possible harm that may occur
    d. explanation of theropeutic alternatives to the proposed ~~protoc~~ procedure, risks of doing nothing.
14. The nurse's signature witnessing the consent means nurse provided info about ask/alternatives of a particular procedure. the pt appears confident & voluntary signed in agreement.
15. If a patient is harmed as a direct result of a nursing student's actions or lack of action, who is liable?
    Student instructor, hospital/health care, facility & the edu institution
16. When students are employed as nursing assistants or aides when not attending classes, which tasks should they not perform?
    jobs that dont appear in a job description for a nurses aid or assistant
17. Briefly explain the process that a nurse needs to follow when a staffing assignment is unreasonable.
    Student should be brought to nursing supervisions attention so that the needed help can be obtained, needs to be documented
18. What is the nurse's responsibility with physicians' orders?
    nurses obligated to follow physicans orders unless they believe that the orders are in error, violate policy or would harm pt. ask for clarification if needed.
19. One of the most frequently litigated issues is whether the nurse if the nurse kept the dr informed of the patients condition & document adequately.
20. If a verbal order is necessary, it should be written out and Signed by the physician within 24 hours.

Legal Issues in Nursing Practice

21. Describe the two federal acts that control the manufacture, distribution, and sale of food, medications, and therapeutic devices in Canada.
    a. food & drugs act (1985)
    b. controlled drug & Substances act (1996)
22. What is a nurse obligated to do when care is requested that is contrary to the nurse's personal values?
    provide appropriate care until alternate care arrangements are made
23. What must a nurse do whenever confidential health care information is requested by a third party?
    ask the patient if its ok, they need to sign a release to confidentiality form
24. Bill C-14 permitted physicians and nurse practitioners to provide medical assistance in dying to patients in what two ways?
25. Describe the function of an *advance directive* for health care.
    A mechanism enabling a mentally competent person to plan for a time when he/she may lack the mental capicty to make medical treatment decisions
26. Differentiate an *advance directive* from a *living will*.
    A living will is a document in which the person makes an anticipatory refusal of life-prolonging measures during a future state of mental incompetence
27. Describe the two forms that an advance directive assumes.
    a. instructional directive (person makes descions)
    b. proxy directive (appoints someone to make decisions)
28. Every province and territory has human tissue legislation that provides for both live donor and post mordem (cadamer) of tissues and organs.
29. What is true about the rights of patients admitted to a psychiatric unit on a voluntary basis?
    they should be treated the same as involuntary

Copyright © 2019 Elsevier Canada, a division of Reed Elsevier Canada, Ltd.

30. Briefly explain the purpose of public health legislation.

directed toward the prevention, treatment & suppression of communicable disease, also to report abuse or neglect of other health related issues (they manage it)

31. Describe a nurse's obligation when child abuse or neglect is witnessed or suspected.

must be reported - both witnessed or suspected, to child protection agencies

32. *Risk management* is

a system of ensuring appropriate nursing care by identifying potential hazards & preventing harm from occurring

33. Name a tool used by risk managers and discuss its purpose.

incident report (adverse occurance report) filled by nurse if an error occurs (ex wrong med)

34. Risk management includes documentation. It should be:

a. thorough (facts only)

b. accurate

c. performed in a timely manner w/in a hour

REVIEW QUESTIONS

Select the appropriate answer and cite the rationale for choosing that particular answer.

1. A nurse fails to provide appropriate care while a patient is in restraints and the patient dies. In an ensuing lawsuit, the nurse's actions would be assessed against which of the following?
   a. The practice of an expert nurse
   b. The condition of the patient prior to application of restraints
   c. Whether or not the nurse followed the physician's orders
   d. What a nurse with similar credentials would do in the same setting

Answer:_______________ Rationale:_______________

2. Which of the following is an example of an *unintentional tort*?
   a. Assault
   b. Battery
   c. Invasion of privacy
   d. Negligence

Answer:_______________ Rationale:_______________

3. As a nurse, witnessing a patient's signature on a consent form verifies which of the following? *(Select all that apply.)*
   a. The signature of the patient is authentic.
   b. The patient is fully informed about a medical action.
   c. The patient is consenting voluntarily to a medical action.
   d. The patient has no questions about the medical action to which the patient is consenting.

Answer:_______________ Rationale:_______________

4. Inserting an intravenous line against a patient's wishes could be considered an example of which type of liability?
   a. False imprisonment
   b. Assault
   c. Battery
   d. Negligence

Answer:_______________ Rationale:_______________

Copyright © 2019 Elsevier Canada, a division of Reed Elsevier Canada, Ltd.

5. You are caring for a patient who has requested medical assistance in dying, a procedure that you feel goes against your personal values. Which of the following best describes your responsibility to the patient?
   a. Your fiduciary responsibility is to the patient; you could not refuse to assist with the death of the patient.
   b. You could identify prior to assisting with the death that this is contrary to your personal values and ensure that alternative arrangements are made for nursing care.
   c. You could refuse to care for the patient even if alternative arrangements could not be made for care during assisted dying.
   d. Medical assistance in dying is a personal choice of the patient and you are not obligated in any way to assist as a health professional.

Answer:______________ Rationale:______________

____

____

6. For a nurse to be held liable for negligence, which of the following conditions must be satisfied? *(Select all that apply.)*
   a. Harm was intended to the patient.
   b. Harm was done even though it could not be attributed to the nurse's actions.
   c. The nurse owed the patient a duty of care.
   d. Harm occurred because of the nurse's actions.

Answer:______________ Rationale:______________

____

____

7. A patient who expresses suicidal ideation is admitted voluntarily to a psychiatric unit. After 2 days, the patient decides to leave the unit against medical advice, but is physically restrained from doing so by the nursing staff, who believe that the patient may attempt self-harm after leaving the unit. Which of the following liabilities could apply in this case?
   a. Lack of informed consent
   b. False imprisonment
   c. Assault
   d. Invasion of privacy

Answer:______________ Rationale:______________

____

____

8. Which of the following is *not* included in a nursing practice act?
   a. Definition of scope of practice
   b. Educational requirements for nurses
   c. Difference between medical and nursing practice
   d. Guidelines for fines and imprisonment for criminal negligence

Answer:______________ Rationale:______________

____

____

Copyright © 2019 Elsevier Canada, a division of Reed Elsevier Canada, Ltd.

9 Global Health

PRELIMINARY READING

Chapter 9, pages 115–132

COMPREHENSIVE UNDERSTANDING

Global Health

1. Briefly define *global health.*

   Optimal well-being of all humans & a a fundamental mental human right

2. Define *health equity.*

   absences of systematic disparities in health that are systemically associated w/ social advantage/disadvantage

3. What does the *global burden of disease* measure?

   the health of populations at the regional, country, & the subnational level

4. What are the three main foci of the Sustainable Development goals?

   - end poverty in all its forms everywhere
   - reduce inequality within & among
   - ensure access to affordable, reliable, sustainable, modern energy for all

5. Global citizenship is which of the following? *(Select all that apply.)*
   a. A responsibility as citizens to engage in our local, national, and international community
   b. Acting upon social injustices and inequities
   c. Disempowering individuals to participate in decision making
   d. Interconnectedness

Cultural Diversity

6. A fundamental belief of multiculturalism in Canada is that all citizens are equal ________________.

7. The three largest visible minority groups in Canada are South asians, chinese, and black.

8. When an interpreter is used, what actions does the nurse need to take during the appointment?

   - sit in a triangular arrangement (body lang)
   - look at pts when speaking (use you & I)
   - Slow speaking & clear (short sentences)
   - avoid medical jargon & repeat important info

Understanding Cultural Concepts

9. To provide culturally competent care, you must understand cultural concepts. Briefly explain each of the following:

   a. Culture:
   as shared patterns of learned values & behaviors that are transmitted overtime

   b. Ethnicity:
   a group whose members share a social & cultural heritage

   c. Race:
   a common biological attributes, such as skin colour, shared by a group

   d. Cultural pluralism:
   perspective that promotes respect for the right of others to have different beliefs, values & behaviours

   e. Cultural relativism:
   fosters awareness & appreciation of cultural differences

   f. Enculturation:
   Socialization into ones primary culture during childhood

   g. Acculturation:
   adapting to & adopting characteristics of a new culture

   h. Assimilation:
   process whereby a minority group gradually adopts the attitudes & customs of the mainstream culture

   i. Multiculturalism:
   a process whereby many cultures co-exist in society & maintain their cultural difference

Copyright © 2019 Elsevier Canada, a division of Reed Elsevier Canada, Ltd.

Cultural conflicts

10. Define the following terms.

a. *Cultural imposition*:

use of your own values & beliefs as an absolute guide to interpreting pts behaviour & providing services

b. *Ethnocentrism*:

to view your own way of life more valuable than other

c. *Discrimination*:

treating ppl unfairly on the basis of their group membership

d. *Racism*:

Specific actions & an attitude whereby one group exerts power over others on the basis of their skin colour or racial heritage

Historical Development of the Concept of Culture

11. Define the following terms.

a. *Transcultural nursing*:

b. *Culturally congruent care*:

c. *Culturally competent care*:

d. *Cultural awareness*:

beginning step toward understanding there is a difference

12. Compare *cultural humility* and *cultural sensitivity.*

cultural sensitivity makes you aware there are differences whereas humility changes across a lifetime

13. Briefly describe two strategies a nurse can use to achieve cultural self-awareness.

Ask... how do I relate to others of a different cultures. What sterotypes do I hold

14. Define *cultural safety*.

Considering the redistribution of power & resources in a relationship

Cultural Assessment

15. The goal of a *cultural assessment* is

a systemic & comprehensive examination of the cultural care, values, beliefs, & practices of individuals fams & communities

16. Briefly explain how using a cultural assessment model or tool as a guide with a patient can assist with providing culturally competent care.

encourage pts to share stories to reveal how they think & cultural lifestyle they embrace that would be significant to their care

Selected Components of Cultural Assessment

17. Describe the following components of cultural assessment.

a. *Ethnohistory*:

knowledge of a pt country of orgin & its history & ecological contexts is significant to the provision of health care

b. *Social organization*:

cultural groups consist of units of organization delineated by kinship status hierarchy & roles of their members

c. *Socioeconomic status, biocultural ecology, and health risks*:

the identification of health risks related to the enviroment should be assessed on admission of pts

d. *Language and communication*:

linguistic & communication patterns are associated w/ different cultural groups

e. *Religion and spirituality*:

has a major influence on a persons attitudes toward health & illness, pain, suffering & death

f. *Caring beliefs and practices*:

a pt perciption of their ability to control circumstances or factors in the environment

g. *Experience with professional health care*:

all cultures have concepts of past, present & future dimensions of time

Copyright © 2019 Elsevier Canada, a division of Reed Elsevier Canada, Ltd.

Global Health Nursing

18. Nurses need what five types of foundational understanding to care for patients at local and global levels?

interproffesional edu & collaborative practice global health edu, global health competencies for nursing, national & internation organization for global health, implications for nursing

REVIEW QUESTIONS

Select the appropriate answer, and cite the rationale for choosing that particular answer.

1. When providing care to patients with diverse cultural backgrounds, it is imperative for you to recognize which of the following?
   a. Cultural consideration must be put aside if basic needs are in jeopardy.
   b. Generalizations about the behaviour of a particular group may be inaccurate.
   c. Current health standards should determine the acceptability of cultural practices.
   d. People from all cultures can be expected to say what they mean and mean what they say.

Answer: ______________ Rationale: ______________

2. To be effective in meeting various ethnic needs, which of the following does a nurse need to do?
   a. Treat all patients alike
   b. Be aware of patients' cultural differences
   c. Act as if you are comfortable with the patient's behaviour
   d. Avoid asking questions about the patient's cultural background

Answer: ______________ Rationale: ______________

3. To provide culturally competent nursing care, which of the following does a nurse need to do?
   a. Identify the patient's values, attitudes, beliefs, and practices
   b. Make decisions based solely on his or her own assessment of the patient
   c. Not be overly concerned with using knowledge from conceptual or theoretical models
   d. Acknowledge that a patient's response to his or her health is similar among various ethnic groups

Answer: ______________ Rationale: ______________

4. A nurse who has cultural humility would be expected to demonstrate which of the following?
   a. The nurse shows interpersonal respect in action with others.
   b. The nurse demonstrates awareness of cultural practices.
   c. The nurse expects others to behave and think as the nurse does.
   d. The nurse verbalizes understanding of similarities and differences in cultures.

Answer: ______________ Rationale: ______________

5. Which of the following is *not* included in providing culturally competent care to a patient?
   a. Being sensitive and open to a patient's cultural beliefs
   b. Providing opportunities for a patient to discuss his or her views with you
   c. Ensuring that a patient's traditional health care practice is handled separately from current health approaches
   d. Working collaboratively with a patient in making health care decisions

Answer: ______________ Rationale: ______________

Copyright © 2019 Elsevier Canada, a division of Reed Elsevier Canada, Ltd.

10 Indigenous Health

PRELIMINARY READING

Chapter 10, pages 133–156

COMPREHENSIVE UNDERSTANDING

Indigenous Diversity—The Canadian Perspective

1. Indigenous people represent an important and grow ivy group in Canada.

Match the term on the left with the correct definition on the right.

c	2. Indigenous people	a.	Legal term for all Canadian Indigenous persons who are not Inuit
a	3. Indian	b.	Registered under the *Indian Act*
d	4. Métis	c.	Includes First Nations, Métis, and Inuit
f	5. Treaty Indian	d.	Specific cultured entity formed post-contact and precolonization
b	6. Status Indian	e.	Sets out federal regulation of reserves
e	7. *Indian Act*	f.	Status Indian who signed a treaty with the Crown

8. Explain the role of Indigenous interpreters who translate for Indigenous patients.

can understand & translate the language & can also make concepts relevant w/in the cultural realm, interpreting the culture for the health provider

Indigenous History in Canada

9. In 1951, changes to the *Indian Act* lifted bans on tradional practices & ceremonies lifted and women were included in ban demrcracy ____.

10. In 1960, Indigenous people were given the right to vote.

11. Describe how Indigenous people view and practice *holistic health.*

experienced healing & wellbeing through a holistic view of health in which illness & treatment consisted of physical emotional mental & spiritual dimensions

12. Explain *colonialism* and its contribution to *historical trauma.*

the development of institutions & policies by European imperial & Euro-American settler gov towards indigenous peoples

13. Describe four objectives of the *residential schools.*

a. sever the link between identities & culture
b. to eliminate indigenous ppl as a group & to assimilate them into canadian security
c. to avoid the legan & finacial obligations that the federal govt had w/ them
d. to gain control over their lands & resources

14. Identify four ways in which *intergenerational trauma* is experienced by Indigenous people.

a. suicide
b. alcohol or other substances
c. sexual abuse
d. poor diets

15. Define *cultural genocide.*

destruction of those structures & practices that allow the group to continue as a group

16. Identify four calls to action arising out of the Truth and Reconciliation Commission, including one that specifically refers to medical and nursing education.

a. Child welfare
b. justic
c. edu
d. language rights

17. The *Sixties Scoop* refers to a situation in which Indigenous children were apprehended from reservations & indigenous families in order to save them.

Copyright © 2019 Elsevier Canada, a division of Reed Elsevier Canada, Ltd.

18. Research has indicated that children who were removed from their homes and placed with non-Indigenous families were abused/neglected and eventually left their adopted families

19. Data from 2010 indicate that child poverty is decreasing among Indigenous children. True or False?

20. Explain the reasons for the negative impacts of incarceration on Indigenous people.

removes them from their families & communities, gateways, to gateways to gang life (youth), racism

Cultural Orientations

21. Describe how the circle symbolizes the *Indigenous worldview.*

it represents the interconnectiveness of all beings

22. Identify the four aspects of health that need to be in balance, according to *Indigenous health.*

a. emotional
b. phyiscal
c. Spiritual
d. mental

Nursing Considerations and Indigenous Health

23. Identify three different *determinants of health.*

a. proximal determinants of health
b. intermediate determinants of health
c. distal determinants of health

24. Identify factors that contribute to the prevalence of diabetes among Indigenous peoples.

genetic susuptibility, transitioning from active to sedentary, intake, of & diet high in Sugar, fats & salts, inequalities, social, political, economical detriments of health

25. HIV/AIDS has led Indigenous communities to organize culturally and become active resulting in culturally safe programs and edu initiatives that resonate with indigenous youth, including two Spirited youth.

26. Two types of cancer that are particularly found among the circumpolar Inuit population are lung cancer and breast cancer.

27. Identify eight factors that may contribute to the high rate of COPD among Inuit and First Nations peoples.

a. exposure to enviromental containments
b. housing conditions, mold, poor ventilation
c. lower levels of edu
d. poor nutrition
e. poverty
f. remote locations
g. childhood exposure of cig smoke
h.

28. Indigenous women evidenced lack of awareness of their own risk factors for cardiovascular disease, which was attributed to a focus on others as the family care giver, often in chaotic and busy circumstances and often with lack of support from men in the fam & community.

29. Hearing loss, related to the incidence of otitis media, has been reported as high as 44% for adult Inuit and as high as 39% for adult First Nations people.

30. arthritis is the most common chronic disorder among Indigenous Canadians.

31. Identify at least four effective approaches to promoting nonaddictive health.

indignesous values, perspectives & knowledge, info on traditional diet, trad indigenous activities & healing practices

Copyright © 2019 Elsevier Canada, a division of Reed Elsevier Canada, Ltd.

REVIEW QUESTIONS

Select the appropriate answer, and cite the rationale for choosing that particular answer.

1. A young Indigenous woman is admitted to hospital following a serious motor vehicle accident. On admission to the unit, the nurse notices that the family has attached a medicine pouch to the young woman's gown, close to her heart. The nurse needs to remove the gown periodically to provide care and wonders if the pouch can be removed. Which of the following actions would suggest that the nurse is demonstrating respect for the patient and family and understanding of the importance of spirituality?
   a. Pins the medicine pouch to the bulletin board near the head of the bed so that it is safe
   b. Ties the medicine pouch to the railing where the young woman can see it, if alert
   c. Asks the family if the pouch can be removed temporarily to a different location
   d. Ties the medicine pouch to a different body location (e.g., the patient's toe)

Answer: ______________ Rationale: ______________

____

____

2. The changes to the *Indian Act* in 1951 were an important step toward recognizing which of the following?
   a. Right of the Indigenous people to self-govern
   b. Removal of requirement for Indigenous children to attend residential schools
   c. Legal assertion of Indigenous people to land rights
   d. Significant role of women in Indigenous self-governance

Answer: ______________ Rationale: ______________

____

____

3. Which of the following describes Indigenous people? *(Select all that apply.)*
   a. Most live on reserves in rural areas
   b. Rate of population growth is higher than for non-Indigenous population
   c. Indigenous population in Canada is younger than the non-Indigenous population
   d. Each indigenous group has an identifiable, unique language and a specific cultural practice

Answer: ______________ Rationale: ______________

____

____

4. Which of the following would be an example of structural racism?
   a. Suicide rates for children of survivors are higher than for survivors themselves
   b. Addiction is a way to deal with the effects of post-traumatic stress disorder
   c. Sexual abuse is common in many Indigenous communities
   d. Health and justice services for Indigenous peoples are characterized by delay and disruption

Answer: ______________ Rationale: ______________

____

____

5. Which of the following would be a priority when beginning an assessment of the health needs of an Indigenous person on the first health visit?
   a. Provide space and privacy for spiritual practices
   b. Take time to find out who the person is and the person's needs
   c. Explain the purpose of your assessment strategies
   d. Use a systematic approach to the health interview

Answer: ______________ Rationale: ______________

____

____

Copyright © 2019 Elsevier Canada, a division of Reed Elsevier Canada, Ltd.

11 Nursing Leadership, Management, and Collaborative Practice

PRELIMINARY READING

Chapter 11, pages 157–173

COMPREHENSIVE UNDERSTANDING

1. Define *collaborative practice.*

Leadership Theories

2. Explain *transformational leadership.*

Management and leadership roles for nurses

3. Describe how nurses can transform health systems.

4. Define *continuity of care.*

5. Briefly explain the following delivery systems.

   a. *Functional nursing*:

   b. *Team nursing*:

   c. *Primary nursing*:

   d. *Case management*:

   e. *Collaborative practice*:

6. Briefly explain the following management structures.

   a. Centralized management:

   b. Decentralized or participatory management:

   c. Matrix:

7. Identify the responsibilities of a nurse manager in a decentralized management structure.

8. Briefly explain responsibility and accountability within the context of decentralized management.

   a. *Responsibility*:

   b. *Accountability*:

Copyright © 2019 Elsevier Canada, a division of Reed Elsevier Canada, Ltd.

9. The nurse manager nurtures and supports staff involvement through the following approaches. Briefly explain each.

   a. Nursing practice or professional shared governance councils:

   b. Interprofessional collaboration:

   c. Staff communication:

   d. Learning organization:

10. Give an example of how a student nurse may be involved as a member of a learning organization in a practice setting.

11. Summarize each of the following leadership and management competencies a student nurse may develop for entry into registered nurse (RN) practice.

   a. Clinical decisions:

   b. Priority setting:

   c. Time management:

   d. Evaluation:

12. Define *delegation*.

13. What institutional documents guide the tasks and activities that can be delegated to UCPs?

14. What is the difference between *delegation* and *assignment*?

15. Identify four points to be considered when assessing whether or not to delegate.

   a.

   b.

   c.

   d.

Quality Care and Patient Safety

16. Where does a definition of quality begin?

17. Define each of the elements of quality nursing practice.

   a. *Professional standards*:

   b. *Care and best practice guidelines*:

   c. *Nurse-sensitive outcomes*:

18. Give an example of a *nurse-sensitive outcome*.

19. Define *patient safety*.

Copyright © 2019 Elsevier Canada, a division of Reed Elsevier Canada, Ltd.

20. What seven core elements for all health care providers are important for developing a culture of patient safety?

______, ______,
______, ______,
______, ______,
______, ______,
______, ______,
______, ______,
______, ______

Leadership Skills for Nursing Students

21. Identify seven ways in which nursing students can learn nursing leadership.

______, ______,
______, ______,
______, ______,
______, ______,
______, ______,
______, ______,
______, ______

REVIEW QUESTIONS

Select the appropriate answer, and cite the rationale for choosing that particular answer.

1. Primary nursing refers to which of the following?
   a. Nurses who work with physicians in primary care
   b. Nurses who hold management positions
   c. Placing RNs in a continuous, direct-care role with patients in health care organizations
   d. Nursing carried out in primary health care

Answer: ______ Rationale: ______

2. A student nurse practicing in a collaborative practice model would demonstrate all but which of the following?
   a. Understanding the patient and family perspective
   b. Recognizing other team members for their contribution
   c. Assuming primary responsibility for planning, implementation, follow-up, and evaluation
   d. Developing listening skills and being aware of personal motivation

Answer: ______ Rationale: ______

3. Decentralized management is best described as which of the following?
   a. Care decisions being made by a manager in another location
   b. Situations in which there is a lack of coordination of care
   c. Situations in which staff overrule the decisions made by managers
   d. Situations in which decision making occurs at the staff level

Answer: ______ Rationale: ______

4. A UCP has a job description that outlines what activities he or she can perform while working at a particular institution. The job description has outlined which of the following?
   a. The UCP's autonomy
   b. The authority of the UCP
   c. The UCP's responsibility
   d. The accountability of the UCP

Answer: ______ Rationale: ______

5. Which of the following is *not* a purpose for delegation?
   a. Improves efficiency
   b. Provides job enrichment
   c. Transfers accountability for patient care
   d. Improves utilization of health care providers

Answer: ______ Rationale: ______

6. A nurse manager who inspires through a vision of excellence in care and who regularly consults with and acknowledges the strength of the team could best be described as having which one of the following leadership styles?
   a. Transformational
   b. Centralized
   c. Emotionally intelligent
   d. Authentic

Answer: ______ Rationale: ______

Copyright © 2019 Elsevier Canada, a division of Reed Elsevier Canada, Ltd.

12 Critical Thinking in Nursing Practice

PRELIMINARY READING

Chapter 12, pages 174–186

COMPREHENSIVE UNDERSTANDING

Critical decision making separates professional nurses from technical or ancillary personnel.

Critical Thinking Defined

1. Define *critical thinking.*

2. To think critically, you must be able to examine the following within the context of the situation.
   a.
   b.
   c.
   d.
   e.

3. Identify the core critical thinking skills that apply to nursing.
   a.
   b.
   c.
   d.
   e.
   f.

A Critical Thinking Model for Clinical Decision Making

4. Summarize the critical thinking model and list its five components.
   a.
   b.
   c.
   d.
   e.

Levels of Critical Thinking in Nursing

5. Three levels of critical thinking in nursing have been identified. Briefly describe each.
   a. Basic:
   b. Complex:
   c. Commitment:

Components of Critical Thinking in Nursing

6. Identify what constitutes a nurse's knowledge base.

7. Identify the ways in which critical thinking is developed through experience.

Critical Thinking Competencies

8. Define *scientific method.*

Copyright © 2019 Elsevier Canada, a division of Reed Elsevier Canada, Ltd.

9. List the five steps of the scientific method.
   a. ______
   b. ______
   c. ______
   d. ______
   e. ______

10. Define *problem solving.*

______

______

11. Define *decision making.*

______

______

12. Explain the process that an individual needs to go through to make a decision.

______

______

______

13. Explain the process of *diagnostic reasoning.*

______

______

______

14. As you gain experience, you will increase your ability to identify ______ and to differentiate ______ ______ and those that are ______ ______.

15. Cite some examples of how nurses make decisions about their patients.

______

______

______

16. The nursing process is a systematic and comprehensive approach for nursing care. List the five steps of the nursing process.
   a. ______
   b. ______
   c. ______
   d. ______
   e. ______

Developing Critical Thinking Skills

17. Explain how *case-based learning* develops critical thinking skills.

______

______

18. Explain how *reflective writing* develops critical thinking skills.

______

______

______

19. What is a concept map?

______

______

______

Critical Thinking Synthesis

20. Briefly explain how the nursing process and the critical thinking model work together.

______

______

______

REVIEW QUESTIONS

Select the appropriate answer, and cite the rationale for choosing that particular answer.

1. Clinical decision making requires a nurse to do which of the following? *(Select all that apply.)*
   a. Improve a patient's health
   b. Establish and weigh criteria in deciding the best choice of therapy for a patient
   c. Follow the physician's orders for patient care
   d. Standardize care for the patient
   e. Know the patient

Answer:______ Rationale:______

______

______

2. Which of the following is *not* one of the five steps of the nursing process?
   a. Planning
   b. Evaluation
   c. Hypothesis testing
   d. Assessment

Answer:______ Rationale:______

______

______

Copyright © 2019 Elsevier Canada, a division of Reed Elsevier Canada, Ltd.

3. Gathering, verifying, and communicating data about the patient to establish a database is an example of which component of the nursing process?
   a. Assessment
   b. Planning
   c. Evaluation
   d. Nursing diagnosis
   e. Implementation

Answer:______________ Rationale:______________
____
____

4. Completing nursing actions necessary for accomplishing a care plan is an example of which component of the nursing process?
   a. Assessment
   b. Planning
   c. Evaluation
   d. Nursing diagnosis
   e. Implementation

Answer:______________ Rationale:______________
____
____

Copyright © 2019 Elsevier Canada, a division of Reed Elsevier Canada, Ltd.

13 Nursing Assessment, Diagnosis, and Planning

PRELIMINARY READING

Chapter 13, pages 187–211

COMPREHENSIVE UNDERSTANDING

1. The nursing process comprises the following five steps: ________, ________, ________, ________, and ________.

Critical Thinking Approach to Assessment

2. Nursing assessment is the systematic process of ________ and ________ from a primary source (the client) and secondary sources (e.g., the family, health providers, and client record) and ________ as a basis for developing ________ ________.

3. Identify the purpose of the assessment.

4. How does critical thinking enhance assessment?

Assessment

5. What four sociocultural variables are included in assessment?

6. A systems review should always begin with ________ and ________ and follow with ________.

7. Define each of the following:
   a. *Subjective data*:
   b. *Objective data*:

8. Identify the types of information a client can provide.
   a.
   b.
   c.
   d.
   e.

9. Families can be an important secondary source of information about the client's health status. Give an example.

10. What four types of information are health care team members able to provide about a client?
    a.
    b.
    c.
    d.

11. By reviewing medical records, you can find information about a client's ________, as well as ________ and ________ test results, current physical findings, and ________ plan.

12. A nurse's ability to make an assessment will develop as he or she ________ and ________ propositions, questions, and principle-based or standard-based expectations.

Copyright © 2019 Elsevier Canada, a division of Reed Elsevier Canada, Ltd.

13. During an interview, nurses have the opportunity to:
    a. ______
    b. ______
    c. ______
    d. ______
    e. ______

14. Describe the phases of the interview.
    a. ______
    b. ______
    c. ______

15. How are closed-ended questions used in an interview?

______

16. When conducting an assessment with a client who is Indigenous, on what should a beginning nurse focus?

______

17. When documenting health history findings, the nurse provides a database that is ______.

18. Identify some nonverbal behaviours that a nurse may observe during assessment.

______

19. Discuss the importance of validation.

______

20. After collecting and validating subjective and objective data and interpreting the data, the nurse organizes the information into meaningful clusters. Data analysis involves recognizing ______.

21. What is the basic rule of documentation?

______

Nursing Diagnosis

22. Define *nursing diagnosis.*

______

23. Define *medical diagnosis.*

______

24. Define *collaborative problem.*

______

25. What are the five purposes of nursing diagnostic statements?

______

Critical Thinking and the Nursing Diagnostic Process

26. The diagnostic process includes ______, ______, and ______.

27. Defining characteristics of the nursing diagnostic process are ______.

28. Briefly explain the four types of nursing diagnoses identified by NANDA International.
    a. Actual nursing diagnosis: ______
    b. Risk nursing diagnosis: ______
    c. Health promotion nursing diagnosis: ______
    d. Wellness nursing diagnosis: ______

Copyright © 2019 Elsevier Canada, a division of Reed Elsevier Canada, Ltd.

29. Nursing diagnoses are stated in a two-part format: the ______________ followed by a ______________.

30. The diagnostic label of the nursing diagnosis is approved by ______________ and describes ______________.

31. The related factors of the nursing diagnosis are ______________. It is associated with ______________ and can be changed through ______________.

32. Risk factors are ______, ______, ______, ______, or ______________ that increase the vulnerability of ______________ to an unhealthful event.

Concept Mapping for Nursing Diagnosis

33. What does a concept map show?

____

Sources of Diagnostic Errors

34. Identify five ways in which diagnostic errors can be made during interpretation of data.

____

____

____

____

____

Nursing Diagnosis: Application to Care Planning

35. Nursing diagnosis is a mechanism for ______________ for clients.

Planning

36. Explain how planning is utilized in nursing.

____

____

Establishing Priorities

37. Priorities are classified as high, intermediate, or low. Explain what is meant by each priority.

a. High priority:

____

____

b. Intermediate priority:

____

____

c. Low priority:

____

____

Critical Thinking in Establishing Goals and Expected Outcomes

38. Define the following:

a. *Client-centred goal*: ______________

____

b. *Short-term goal*: ______________

____

c. *Long-term goal*: ______________

____

d. *Expected outcome*: ______________

____

e. *Nursing-sensitive client outcome*: ______________

____

39. Define and give an example of each of the seven guidelines to follow when writing goals and expected outcomes.

a. *Client goal or outcome*: ______________

____

b. *Singular*: ______________

____

c. *Observable*: ______________

____

d. *Measurable*: ______________

____

e. *Time-limited*: ______________

____

f. *Mutual*: ______________

____

g. *Realistic*: ______________

____

Copyright © 2019 Elsevier Canada, a division of Reed Elsevier Canada, Ltd.

Written Plans of Care

40. A written nursing care plan includes ____________, ____________, and ____________.

41. Briefly explain a critical pathway.

____

____

Consulting with Other Health Care Professionals

42. Consultation occurs most often during ____________.

REVIEW QUESTIONS

Select the appropriate answer, and cite the rationale for choosing that particular answer.

1. In most circumstances, the best source of information for nursing assessment of the adult client is which of the following?
   a. Nursing literature
   b. Physician
   c. Client
   d. Medical record

Answer:____________ Rationale:____________

____

____

2. Reviewing the client's medical record to obtain baseline data about the client's response to illness occurs during which phase of the nursing process?
   a. Planning
   b. Nursing diagnosis
   c. Evaluation
   d. Assessment

Answer:____________ Rationale:____________

____

____

3. Which of the following accurately defines a nursing diagnosis?
   a. It is a statement of a client response to a health problem that requires nursing intervention.
   b. It identifies health problems within the domain of nursing.
   c. It is derived from the physician's history and physical examination.
   d. It is not changed during the course of a client's hospitalization.

Answer:____________ Rationale:____________

____

____

4. Mr. Margauz, a 52-year-old business executive, is admitted to the coronary care unit. During his admission interview, he denies chest pain or shortness of breath. His pulse and blood pressure are normal. He appears tense and does not want you to leave his bedside. When questioned, he states that he is very nervous. At this moment, which nursing diagnosis is the most appropriate?
   a. Alteration in comfort, chest pain
   b. Alteration in bowel elimination related to restricted mobility
   c. High risk for altered cardiac output related to heart attack
   d. Anxiety related to critical care unit admission

Answer:____________ Rationale:____________

____

____

5. "The client will remain free from infection throughout hospitalization" appears on the nursing care plan for an immunosuppressed client. This is an example of which of the following?
   a. Long-term goal
   b. Short-term goal
   c. Nursing diagnosis
   d. Expected outcome

Answer:____________ Rationale:____________

____

____

Copyright © 2019 Elsevier Canada, a division of Reed Elsevier Canada, Ltd.

14 Implementing and Evaluating Nursing Care

PRELIMINARY READING

Chapter 14, pages 212–232

COMPREHENSIVE UNDERSTANDING

1. ______________ and ______________ ______ follow assessment, diagnosis, and planning in the nursing process.

Implementation

2. Define the fourth step in the nursing process.

3. Define the following terms related to implementation.

   a. *Direct care*: ______________

   b. *Indirect care*: ______________

   c. *Nursing intervention*: ______________

Types of Nursing Interventions

4. Define the following terms.

   a. *Independent nursing intervention*: ______________

   b. *Dependent nursing intervention*: ______________

   c. *Collaborative intervention*: ______________

Selection of Interventions

5. Identify the six factors to be considered when choosing an intervention.

6. List the domains of practice included in the Nursing Intervention Classification (NIC) model.

Critical Thinking in Implementation

7. Briefly explain the activities for making decisions during implementation.

   a. ______________

   b. ______________

   c. ______________

   d. ______________

Standard Nursing Interventions

8. Define the following terms.

   a. *Medical directive or standing order*: ______________

   b. *Clinical practice guideline or protocol*: ______________

Implementation Process

9. Briefly explain the five preparatory activities for implementation of safe and effective care.

   a. Reassessing the client: ______________

   b. Reviewing and revising the existing nursing care plan: ______________

Copyright © 2019 Elsevier Canada, a division of Reed Elsevier Canada, Ltd.

c. Organizing resources and care delivery: ______

d. Anticipating and preventing complications: ______

e. Implementation skills: ______

Direct Care

10. Provide an example of when RN/LPN/RPN scopes of practice overlap but roles differ in care. ______

11. Define *activities of daily living* (ADLs). ______

12. *Instrumental activities of daily living* (IADLs) include ______.

13. *Physical care techniques* include ______.

14. *Controlling for adverse reactions* includes ______.

15. *Life-saving measures* are ______.

16. *Counselling* is ______.

17. The *focus of teaching* is ______.

18. *Preventive nursing actions* are ______.

Indirect Care

19. Provide an example of indirect care. ______

Achieving Client-Centred Goals

20. Effective discharge planning and teaching for clients and families should be initiated at ______.

Evaluation

21. Identify two components of evaluation.
    a. ______
    b. ______

Critical Thinking and Evaluation

22. Explain how the utilization of critical thinking in the analysis of findings contributes to evaluation. ______

The Evaluation Process

23. Identify the five elements of the evaluation process.
    a. ______
    b. ______
    c. ______
    d. ______
    e. ______

24. Define *standard of care.* ______

25. Define *outcome.* ______

26. List the purposes of the Nursing Outcomes Classification.
    a. ______
    b. ______
    c. ______

27. Define *evaluative measures.* ______

28. Briefly explain the following parts of the evaluative process.
    a. Care plan revision: ______
    b. Discontinuing a care plan: ______

Copyright © 2019 Elsevier Canada, a division of Reed Elsevier Canada, Ltd.

c. Modifying a care plan: ______________________________

____

____

Conclusion

29. Through continuous evaluation of care, nurses play a key role in ______________________________.

Using the Nursing Process as a Guide for Exam Preparation and Test Taking

30. Common words in the stem or question of an exam item help to ______________________________.

REVIEW QUESTIONS

Select the appropriate answer, and cite the rationale for choosing that particular answer.

1. Evaluation is best described by which of the following? *(Select all that apply.)*
   a. Begun immediately before the patient's discharge
   b. Involves assessment skills and techniques
   c. Necessary only if the physician orders it
   d. An integrated, ongoing nursing care activity
   e. Performed primarily by nurses in the quality-assurance department

Answer: __________ Rationale: ______________________________

2. Measuring the patient's response to nursing interventions and his or her progress toward achieving goals occurs during which phase of the nursing process?
   a. Planning
   b. Nursing diagnosis
   c. Evaluation
   d. Assessment

Answer: __________ Rationale: ______________________________

3. When a client-centred goal has not been met within the projected time frame, the most appropriate action would be which of the following?
   a. Rewrite the plan, using different interventions
   b. Continue with the same plan until the goal is met
   c. Repeat the nursing process sequence to discover needed changes
   d. Conclude the goal was inappropriate or unrealistic and eliminate it from the plan

Answer: __________ Rationale: ______________________________

4. Which of the following is not true of standing orders? *(Select all that apply.)*
   a. Standing orders are commonly found in critical care and community health settings.
   b. Standing orders are approved and signed by the health care provider before implementation.
   c. With standing orders, nurses have the legal protection to intervene appropriately in the client's best interest.
   d. With standing orders, the nurse is not required to determine if the intervention is appropriate at the time of care.

Answer: __________ Rationale: ______________________________

5. A client has been newly diagnosed with type 1 diabetes. The nurse shows the client how to inject insulin. Which intervention activity is being utilized by the nurse?
   a. Life-saving
   b. Teaching
   c. Managing
   d. Counselling

Answer: __________ Rationale: ______________________________

6. A client comes to the family clinic for birth control. The nurse obtains a health history and performs a pelvic examination and Pap smear. The nurse is acting in accordance with which of the following?
   a. Clinical protocol or best practice guideline
   b. Standing order
   c. Nursing care plan
   d. Dependent nursing intervention

Answer: __________ Rationale: ______________________________

Copyright © 2019 Elsevier Canada, a division of Reed Elsevier Canada, Ltd.

15 Documenting and Reporting

PRELIMINARY READING

Chapter 15, pages 233–253

COMPREHENSIVE UNDERSTANDING

1. What is *documentation*?

____

____

____

Purposes of Medical Records

Match the term on the left with the correct definition on the right.

2. ____ communication
3. ____ legal documentation
4. ____ funding and resource management
5. ____ education
6. ____ research
7. ____ auditing and monitoring

a. Objective, ongoing reviews to determine the degree to which quality improvement standards are met
b. Learning about the nature of an illness and the response of the patient
c. Means by which patient needs and progress, individual therapies, patient education, and planning are conveyed to others in the health care team
d. Gathering statistical data about clinical disorders, complications, therapies, recovery, and death
e. Describes exactly what happened to the patient and follows agency standards
f. Supports how and when resources are used in patient care

The Shift to Electronic Documentation

8. Define each of the following:

a. *Electronic medical record*:

____

____

b. *Electronic health record*:

____

____

9. Identify the unique feature of an *EHR*.

____

Interprofessional Communication within the Medical Record

10. Four attributes of patient information are

_______________, _______________,

_______________, and _______________.

Confidentiality

11. Identify who has access to patient information.

____

12. Give five examples of how students can breach confidentiality.

____

____

____

____

____

13. Define *PIPEDA*.

____

____

Interprofessional Communication within the Health Team

14. Caregivers use a variety of ways to exchange information about patients. Briefly explain the following:

a. Patient record or chart:

____

____

____

b. Reports:

____

____

____

Copyright © 2019 Elsevier Canada, a division of Reed Elsevier Canada, Ltd.

Guidelines for Quality Documentation and Reporting

15. High-quality documentation and reporting have six important characteristics: They are factual, accurate, complete, current, organized, and they comply with standards set by Accreditation Canada and by provincial or territorial regulatory bodies. Explain each characteristic.

    a. Factual:

    b. Accurate:

    c. Complete:

    d. Current:

    e. Organized:

    f. Compliant with standards:

Methods of Documentation

16. Narrative documentation is a storylike format that documents information specific to patient conditions and nursing care. What are the disadvantages of this style?

    a.

    b.

    c.

17. *Problem-oriented medical records* place emphasis on the patient's problems. The method corresponds to the nursing process and facilitates communication of patient needs. Explain the following major sections of the problem-oriented medical record.

    a. Database:

    b. Problem list:

    c. Care plan:

    d. Progress notes:

18. Define the acronyms, and briefly explain the forms of documentation of the problem-oriented medical record.

    a. *SOAP or SOAPIE notes*:

    b. *PIE format*:

    c. *Focus charting or DAR*:

19. Briefly explain the following forms of documentation.

    a. Source records:

    b. Charting by exception:

    c. Critical pathways or care maps:

Common Record-Keeping Forms

20. Briefly explain the following formats used for record keeping.

    a. Admission nursing history forms:

    b. Flow sheets and graphic records:

    c. Patient care summary or Kardex:

Copyright © 2019 Elsevier Canada, a division of Reed Elsevier Canada, Ltd.

d. Standardized care plans:

e. Discharge summary forms:

Acuity Rating Systems

21. Explain the purpose of *acuity ratings*.

Home Health Care Documentation

22. Documentation in the home health care system has implications different from those it has in other areas of nursing. List two primary differences.
    a.
    b.

Documentation in the Long-Term Health Care Setting

23. Because residents are stable, documentation is done using ______________, and assessment may be done only ______________.

Documenting Communication with Providers and Unique Events

24. Documentation regarding a telephone call *to* a health care provider includes ______________, ______________, ______________, ______________, ______________, and ______________.

25. List the guidelines the nurse should follow when receiving telephone orders from physicians.
    a.
    b.
    c.
    d.
    e.
    f.

26. Identify the eight major areas to include in a *change-of-shift* report.
    a.
    b.
    c.
    d.
    e.
    f.
    g.
    h.

27. List the nine major information areas in a *transfer report*.
    a.
    b.
    c.
    d.
    e.
    f.
    g.
    h.
    i.

28. Define *SBAR* or *I-SBAR-R*.

29. Describe the purpose of an *incident report*.

Information Management in Health Care

30. Define *health informatics*.

31. Define each of the following:
    a. *Clinical information system*:
    b. *Computerized provider order entry*:
    c. *Clinical decision support system*:
    d. *Nursing clinical information system*:

Copyright © 2019 Elsevier Canada, a division of Reed Elsevier Canada, Ltd.

REVIEW QUESTIONS

Select the appropriate answer, and cite the rationale for choosing that particular answer.

1. What is the primary purpose of a patient's medical record?
   a. To satisfy the requirements of accreditation agencies
   b. To communicate accurate, timely information about the patient
   c. To provide validation for hospital charges
   d. To provide the nurse with a defence against malpractice

Answer:_______________ Rationale:_______________

____

____

2. Which of the following is charted according to the six guidelines for quality recording?
   a. "Respirations rapid; lung sounds clear."
   b. "Was depressed today."
   c. "Crying. States she doesn't want visitors to see her like this."
   d. "Had a good day. Up and about in room."

Answer:_______________ Rationale:_______________

____

____

3. Which of the following best describes a *change-of-shift report*?
   a. Two or more nurses always visit all patients to review their plan of care.
   b. Nurses should exchange judgements they have made about patient attitudes.
   c. The nurse should identify nursing diagnoses and clarify patient priorities.
   d. Patient information is communicated from a nurse on a sending unit to a nurse on a receiving unit.

Answer:_______________ Rationale:_______________

____

____

4. What is an *incident report*?
   a. A legal claim against a nurse for negligent nursing care
   b. A summary report of all falls occurring on a nursing unit
   c. A report of an event inconsistent with the routine care of a patient
   d. A report of a nurse's behaviour submitted to the hospital administration

Answer:_______________ Rationale:_______________

____

____

5. If an error is made while recording, what should you do?
   a. Erase it or scratch it out
   b. Obtain a new nurse's note and rewrite the entries
   c. Leave a blank space in the note
   d. Draw a single line through the error, and initial it

Answer:_______________ Rationale:_______________

____

____

Copyright © 2019 Elsevier Canada, a division of Reed Elsevier Canada, Ltd.

16 Nursing Informatics and Canadian Nursing Practice

PRELIMINARY READING

Chapter 16, pages 254–270

COMPREHENSIVE UNDERSTANDING

1. Define *nursing informatics (NI)*.

___

___

Nursing Informatics and the Canadian Health Care System

2. Describe the purpose of the *electronic health record.*

___

___

___

3. Early definitions of NI focused on ______ ______ and ______ ______; more recent definitions focus on ______ as an ______.

4. Define the acronym and describe the evolution of what is now known as *CIHI.*

___

___

___

___

___

___

5. Describe the three components of the mandate of the *Canada Health Infoway.*

___

___

___

Standards and Clinical Interoperability

6. Standards in health care data management refer to the established and formally endorsed coding protocols for all health information, including coding of what aspects of health care delivery?

a. ______

b. ______

c. ______

d. ______

7. Describe the two types of needs that can stimulate the need for a data management standard.

a. Technical needs:

___

___

b. Business needs:

___

___

8. Define *SNOWMED-CT.*

___

___

9. Describe what is meant by a *nursing minimum data set.*

___

___

___

10. *Health Information: Nursing Components (HI:NC)* is composed of five categories of elements. List and describe the five categories.

a. ______

___

b. ______

___

c. ______

___

d. ______

___

e. ______

___

11. Describe the role of the International Council of Nurses in developing the International Classification for Nursing Practice (ICNP®).

___

___

___

___

Copyright © 2019 Elsevier Canada, a division of Reed Elsevier Canada, Ltd.

12. What is the ICNP®, and what is its use?

____

____

____

____

13. ICNP® uses seven axes to capture the core details of nursing practice for coding key nursing data in the electronic health record. Identify the seven axes.

a. ______________________________________

b. ______________________________________

c. ______________________________________

d. ______________________________________

e. ______________________________________

f. ______________________________________

g. ______________________________________

14. What is *C-HOBIC* and what does it report?

____

____

____

____

Canadian Privacy Legislation

15. What are the names of the two federal legislative acts that address the privacy of personal information?

a. ______________________________________

b. ______________________________________

16. Describe three examples of personal health information protected specifically by the *Personal Information Protection and Electronic Documents Act (PIPEDA)*.

a. ______________________________________

b. ______________________________________

c. ______________________________________

Informatics Competencies as a Strategic Direction

17. CNA identified seven key outcomes that are projected to emerge from the *E-Nursing Strategy for Canada* (2006). Describe three of these outcomes.

a. ______________________________________

b. ______________________________________

c. ______________________________________

Clinician Engagement and Informatics Communities

Many Canadian and international health informatics communities exist that offer opportunities for participation, support, educational programs, and networking.

18. The following is a list of important health informatics communities. Describe the role of each organization in influencing NI.

a. CNA:

____

____

____

b. Canadian Nursing Informatics Association:

____

____

____

c. COACH:

____

____

____

REVIEW QUESTIONS

Select the appropriate answer, and cite the rationale for choosing that particular answer.

1. As a new graduate, you have just started a new position and find in orientation that the EHR is often cited. You know from your reading that this refers to which of the following?
   a. Events of health risk
   b. Electronic health record
   c. Entries of the health record
   d. Electronic histogram response

Answer: ____________ Rationale: ______________

____

____

2. Which of the following describes C-HOBIC?
   a. Reports nursing-sensitive outcomes
   b. Enables a longitudinal view of a person's health
   c. Identifies clinical work processes for providers
   d. Transfers the jurisdictional oversight needed for safe transmission of messages

Answer: ____________ Rationale: ______________

____

____

Copyright © 2019 Elsevier Canada, a division of Reed Elsevier Canada, Ltd.

3. Which of the following is *not* a component of an EHR?
   a. Diagnostic images
   b. Drugs dispensed to patient
   c. Provider registry
   d. Coding for nursing contributions to health outcomes

Answer:______________ Rationale:______________
____
____

4. Which of the following is *not* one of the HI:NC categories?
   a. Nursing diagnosis
   b. Patient outcome
   c. Primary nurse identifier
   d. Nursing resource intensity

Answer:______________ Rationale:______________
____
____

5. When patients indicate to you that they are afraid that their health information will not be kept confidential, you correctly respond that all nurses are bound to maintain confidentiality by which of the following? *(Select all that apply.)*
   a. CNA *Code of Ethics*
   b. *PIPEDA*
   c. *Privacy Act*
   d. C-HOBIC

Answer:______________ Rationale:______________
____
____

Copyright © 2019 Elsevier Canada, a division of Reed Elsevier Canada, Ltd.

17 Communication and Relational Practice

PRELIMINARY READING

Chapter 17, pages 271–290

COMPREHENSIVE UNDERSTANDING

1. Communication is a lifelong process. This process enables nurses to communicate with persons who are In some of the most stressful of lifes circumstances.

2. Effective communication between patients and nurses promotes:
   a. interproffesional collab w/ others in the health care team
   b. Ensure that ethical & legal responsibilites & professional practice standards are met
   c. contributes to positive pt. outcomes

Communication and Interpersonal Relationships

3. Define *relational practice.* Guided by conscious participation w/ clients using a # of relational skills

4. Explain each of the following elements of *relational communication.*
   a. *Initiative:* Reaching out & listening
   b. *Authenticity:* Spontaneous & genuine, aware of the in-the-moment experiences
   c. *Mutuality:* Respecting each persons autonomy & valve system, being in synch
   d. *Questioning beyond the surface:* An approach to inquiry that facilitates relationl practice w/in complex circumstankes of haeth & illness

Developing Communication Skills

5. Briefly explain the qualities of critical thinking in relation to the communication process.
   Curiosity, perserverance, creativity, self confidence, indepence, fairness, integrity, & humility, are important when approaching a problem

Levels of Communication

6. Summarize the following communication interactions.
   a. *Intrapersonal communication:* self talk or inner thoughts, comminication that occurs within an individual
   b. *Interpersonal communication:* one-to-one interaction, often occurs face-to-face
   c. *Transpersonal communication:* communication + relation w/in a persons spiritual domain
   d. *Small group communication:* an interaction that occurs when a small group meets & share a common goal
   e. *Public communication:* interaction w/ an audience

Basic Elements of the Communication Process

7. Briefly summarize the following elements of communication.
   a. *Referent:* motivates a person to communicate w/ another, certain cues like: setting, sight, sound, odour, time schedules, emotions, etc

Copyright © 2019 Elsevier Canada, a division of Reed Elsevier Canada, Ltd.

b. *Sender*: The person who encodes & delivers the message

c. *Receiver*: who receives + decodes the message

d. *Message*: The content of the communication

e. *Channels*: means of conveying & receiving messages

f. *Feedback*: The message returned by the receiver

g. *Interpersonal variables*: Characteristics within the sender + reciever that influence communication

h. *Environment*: The setting for sender-reciever info

Forms of Communication

8. Briefly explain the important aspects of verbal communication listed below.

a. Vocabulary: communication is unsuccessful if senders & receivers cannot decode each others words

b. Denotative and connotative meaning: words can have different meanings they need to be selected carefully

c. Pacing: it is important to speak slowly enough to enunciate

d. Intonation: Tone of voice dramatically affects the meaning of a message

e. Clarity and brevity: effective communication is simple, brief & direct, fewer words result in less confusion

f. Timing and relevance: Timing is critical the best time for interaction is when the pt shows interest in communication

9. *Nonverbal communication* includes the use of all 5 senses and refers to trasmission of messages that do not involve the spoken or written word

10. Becoming an astute observer of nonverbal behaviour takes practice, concentration, and sensitivity to others. Briefly explain the following nonverbal behaviours.

a. Personal appearance: physical characteristics facial exp, manner of dress, & grooming & adornments

b. Posture and gait: the way people sit, stand & move, reflects attitudes emotions, self concept & health status

c. Facial expression: Convey emotion

d. Eye contact: Signals readiness to communicate

e. Gestures: emphasize punctuate & clarify spoken word & can communicate volumes when speech is not possible

f. Sounds: communicate thoughts + feelings

g. Personal space: provides people w/ a sense of identity, security & control

11. Identify the zones of personal space.

intimate zone - 0-45 cm
personal zone - 45cm - 1m
Social zone - 1m-4m
public zone - 4m & ig

12. Identify the zones of touch.

Social zone - assess for permission
consent zone - consent needed
vulnerable zone - consent & special care needed
intimate zone - consent & great sensitivity needed

Copyright © 2019 Elsevier Canada, a division of Reed Elsevier Canada, Ltd.

13. Summarize *symbolic communication.*
Verbal + non-verbal sybolism used to convey meaning For ex art, music & dance

14. Define *metacommunication.*
broad term that refers to all factors that influence how a message is perceived by otherss

Professional Nursing Relationships

15. Professional relationships are created through Knowledge, understand of behaviour & communication and commitment to ethical behaviour

16. Acceptance conveys a to hear a message or acknowledge feelings.

17. The nurse–patient relationship is characterized by four goal-directed phases. Explain the phases.
    a. Pre-interaction phase: Review data, talk to other caregivers anticipates issues, plan time for interaction
    b. Orientation phase: Set the tone, observe, assess, prioritize negotiate, sets expectations
    c. Working phase: encourages pt to express feelings + set goals, therapeutic comm
    d. Termination phase: evaluate goal achievements, facilitate smoothe transition for pt to other caregivers

18. Nurses often encourage patients to share personal stories. This is called narrative interactions.

Nurse–family relationships

19. Summarize the principles related to nurse–family relationships.

20. Communication in nurse and interprofessional team relationships is geared toward Team building, facilitating group process, collab, consult, delegation, supervision, leadership + management.

21. Communication within the community occurs through channels such as newsletters, public bulletin boards, radio, tv, electronic info. sites, & social media.

Elements of Professional Communication

22. Briefly explain the following elements of professional communication.
    a. Courtesy: greet & say goodbye to pts & knock before entering their room
    b. Use of names: Addressing by name conveys respect for dignity & unginess
    c. Trustworthiness: being trustworthy means following through on what you say you are going to do
    d. Autonomy and responsibility: Ability to be self directed & independant & accepting responsibility for the outcomes of their actions
    e. Assertiveness: Allows individuals to act in their own best interest w/ out infringing or denying rights

Communication within the Nursing Care Process

23. List the contextual factors that influence communication.
    a. physchological
    b. relational
    c. situational
    d. envirnomental
    e. cultural

24. Identify the psychophysiologic contextual factors that influence communication.
physiological status, emotional status, unmet needs attitudes, valves & beliefs

Copyright © 2019 Elsevier Canada, a division of Reed Elsevier Canada, Ltd.

25. List four environmental contextual factors that influence communication.
    a. privacy level
    b. noise level
    c. comfort + Safety level
    d. distraction level

26. Explain how developmental factors influence communication.
    different age groups have different levels of comm & understanding

27. Describe communication that is considered culturally safe *relational inquiry.*

28. Gender influences communication. Explain how communication differs in regard to gender.
    a. Male:
    b. Female:

29. Identify the primary nursing diagnosis that is utilized when a patient has difficulty communicating.

30. What factors must be considered as you design a responsive approach and nursing care plan?
    a. Motivation
    b.
    c.
    d.
    e.

Implementation

31. Therapeutic communication techniques are specific responses that encourage the expression of feelings and ideas while conveying the nurse's acceptance and respect. Briefly explain the following techniques.
    a. *Active listening*:
    Being attentive to what the pt is saying both verbally & non-verbal
    b. *Sharing observations*:
    c. *Sharing empathy*:
    d. *Sharing hope*:
    e. *Sharing humour*:
    f. *Sharing feelings*:
    g. *Using touch*:
    h. *Using silence*:
    i. *Providing information*:
    j. *Clarifying*:
    k. *Focusing*:
    l. *Paraphrasing*:
    m. *Asking relevant questions*:
    n. *Summarizing*:
    o. *Self-disclosure*:

Copyright © 2019 Elsevier Canada, a division of Reed Elsevier Canada, Ltd.

p. *Confrontation*:

32. Certain communication techniques can hinder or damage professional relationships. These techniques are referred to as *nontherapeutic.* Briefly explain the following nontherapeutic techniques.
   a. Asking personal questions:
   b. Giving personal opinions:
   c. Changing the subject:
   d. Automatic responses:
   e. False reassurance:
   f. Sympathy:
   g. Asking for explanations:
   h. Approval or disapproval:
   i. Defensive responses:
   j. Passive or aggressive responses:
   k. Arguing:

33. Briefly identify the communication techniques to use with the patient who has special needs.
   a. Patients who cannot speak clearly:
   b. Patients who are cognitively impaired:
   c. Patients who are hearing impaired:
   d. Patients who are visually impaired:
   e. Patients who are unresponsive:
   f. Patients who do not speak English:

Evaluation

34. Describe the purpose of a *process recording.*

REVIEW QUESTIONS

Select the appropriate answer, and cite the rationale for choosing that particular answer.

1. *Transpersonal communication* can be defined as which of the following?
   a. Interaction that occurs within a person's spiritual domain
   b. One-to-one interaction between the nurse and the patient
   c. Communication within groups
   d. Self-talk

Answer: ______ Rationale: ______

Copyright © 2019 Elsevier Canada, a division of Reed Elsevier Canada, Ltd.

2. In demonstrating the method for deep-breathing exercises, you place your hands on the patient's abdomen to explain diaphragmatic movement. This technique involves the use of which communication element?
   a. Feedback
   b. Tactile channel
   c. Referent
   d. Message

Answer: ______________ Rationale: ______________

____

____

3. Which statement about nonverbal communication is correct?
   a. It is easy for a nurse to judge the meaning of a patient's facial expression.
   b. The nurse's verbal messages should be reinforced by nonverbal cues.
   c. The physical appearance of the nurse rarely influences nurse–patient interaction.
   d. Words convey meanings that are usually more significant than nonverbal communication.

Answer: ______________ Rationale: ______________

____

____

4. The term referring to all of the relational aspects of a message is called which of the following?
   a. Nonverbal communication
   b. Metacommunication
   c. Connotative meaning
   d. Denotative meaning

Answer: ______________ Rationale: ______________

____

____

5. The referent in the communication process is considered which of the following?
   a. That which motivates the communication
   b. The means of conveying messages
   c. Information shared by the sender
   d. The person who initiates the communication

Answer: ______________ Rationale: ______________

____

____

Copyright © 2019 Elsevier Canada, a division of Reed Elsevier Canada, Ltd.

18 Patient-Centred Care: Interprofessional Collaborative Practice

PRELIMINARY READING

Chapter 18, 291–306

COMPREHENSIVE UNDERSTANDING

1. By focusing on the immediate needs of Mrs. Black, you would neglect the ______________________________.

   Therefore, when we provide care that is ______________________, we must integrate ______________________________.

Knowing

2. Provide an example of each of the following:
   a. *Received knowing*: ______________________________
   b. *Subjective knowing*: ______________________________
   c. *Procedural knowing*: ______________________________
   d. *Constructed knowing*: ______________________________

Professional Patterns of Knowing

3. Describe a limitation of *empiric knowing.*

   ____

4. Define *value.*

   ____

5. Describe the relationship between the Canadian nursing *Code of Ethics* and standards.

   ____

Thinking

6. Thinking is used to gain ______________ into what might be helpful to a patient.

The Nursing Process

7. Identify the four steps outlined by Orlando.
   a. ______________________________
   b. ______________________________
   c. ______________________________
   d. ______________________________

Clinical Judgement Model

8. The four aspects of the Clinical Judgement Model are influenced by the ______________ where the ______________ occurs, the ______________ of ______________, and the ______________ that are developed.

9. Define each of the following:
   a. *Noticing*: ______________________________
   b. *Interpreting*: ______________________________
   c. *Responding*: ______________________________
   d. *Reflecting*: ______________________________

10. Identify four questions that could be asked under *reflecting* in the Clinical Judgement Model that could be used to assess your judgement.
    a. ______________________________
    b. ______________________________
    c. ______________________________
    d. ______________________________

11. Define *role clarification.*

    ____

Copyright © 2019 Elsevier Canada, a division of Reed Elsevier Canada, Ltd.

Interacting

12. Define *interprofessional patient-centred collaborative practice.*

13. Discuss each of the following aspects, identified by Adler et al. (2009), that affect how others receive your message.
    a. Affinity:
    b. Immediacy:
    c. Respect:
    d. Control:

14. Preparing your communication using ______ ______ will help you to ensure that the ______ ______ ______within the parameters that you have shared.

15. Describe *focal role.*

16. Describe *team interdependence.*

17. Identify four elements in *transformative leadership.*
    a.
    b.
    c.
    d.

18. Identify eight steps that can be used to resolve conflict in interprofessional teams.
    a.
    b.
    c.
    d.
    e.
    f.
    g.
    h.

REVIEW QUESTIONS

Select the appropriate answer, and cite the rationale for choosing that particular answer.

1. As a student nurse, you are asked to perform wound care for a recent postoperative client. You want to ensure that you are performing the procedure, using the most up-to-date information, and so you consult your nursing textbook as well as a recent research article before you begin the wound care. Which pattern of knowing are you utilizing in this situation?
   a. Standard of care
   b. Empiric
   c. Aesthetic
   d. Interpreting

Answer: ______ Rationale: ______

2. Role clarification is important to function effectively within interprofessional teams. Which of the following describe aspects of role clarification? *(Select all that apply.)*
   a. You are able to articulate your own role.
   b. You are able to articulate your knowledge and expertise.
   c. You are confident that others on the team can articulate their knowledge and expertise.
   d. You are able to retain control of the team because you are confident in your knowledge and expertise.

Answer: ______ Rationale: ______

3. In an interprofessional client-centred collaborative team, which of the following characterizes the leadership of the team?
   a. Members share leadership and encourage others to lead.
   b. An identified leader seeks out opportunities for the team.
   c. Decisions are made primarily by the leader with some input from the team.
   d. Decisions are made by the team and then communicated to the client.

Answer: ______ Rationale: ______

Copyright © 2019 Elsevier Canada, a division of Reed Elsevier Canada, Ltd.

4. During the initial assessment of a client, you listen for what the patient is sharing about the patient's health journey and observe how the patient tells about the journey. Which of Orlando's steps are you utilizing?
   a. Feeling
   b. Thought
   c. Action
   d. Perception

Answer: _______________ Rationale: _______________
____
____

5. Which aspect of Tanner's Clinical Judgement Model are you employing from question 4?
   a. Narrative interpretation
   b. Responding
   c. Noticing
   d. Reflecting

Answer: _______________ Rationale: _______________
____
____

Copyright © 2019 Elsevier Canada, a division of Reed Elsevier Canada, Ltd.

19 Family Nursing

PRELIMINARY READING

Chapter 19, pages 307–323

COMPREHENSIVE UNDERSTANDING

1. Describe the assumptions that are central to *family nursing.*

   ____

2. Describe the goal of family nursing.

   ____

What Is a Family?

3. The *family* can be defined as a set of __________, as a __________, or as a __________.

Current Trends in the Canadian Family

4. Summarize the various *family forms.*
   a. Traditional nuclear family: __________
   b. Extended family: __________
   c. Step-family: __________
   d. Blended family: __________
   e. Lone-parent family: __________
   f. Family forms: Diversity: __________

5. Identify at least three current trends that challenge the family.
   a. __________
   b. __________
   c. __________

Pregnancy for Teens and Older Moms

6. Explain the following trends and social factors that impact the structure and function of the family.
   a. Domestic roles: __________
   b. Economic status: __________
   c. Indigenous families: __________
   d. Family caregivers: __________

The Family and Health

7. The health of the family is influenced by many factors, such as the following:
   a. __________
   b. __________
   c. __________
   d. __________
   e. __________
   f. __________

Copyright © 2019 Elsevier Canada, a division of Reed Elsevier Canada, Ltd.

8. The crisis-proof, or effective, family is able to integrate the need for stability with the need for growth and change. Explain.

9. Define family *hardiness*.

10. Define family *resiliency*.

Family Nursing Care

11. Identify the four competency domains in the National Education Framework of the Canadian Association of Schools of Nursing that emphasize family nursing.

12. List the three things that nurses should examine when they consider how a health problem or illness affects a family and how a family affects a health problem or illness.
    a.
    b.
    c.

13. Briefly explain the following two focuses proposed for family nursing practice.
    a. Family as *context*:
    b. Family as *patient*:

Assessing the Challenges, Strengths, and Needs of the Family: The Calgary Family Assessment Model

14. Summarize the following three major categories of family life that the Calgary Family Assessment Model offers as a framework for nurses to follow when conducting family assessments.
    a. Structural dimension:
    b. Developmental dimension:
    c. Functional dimension:

Structural assessment

15. Explain these terms.
    a. *Internal structure*:
    b. *External structure*:
    c. *Context*:

16. Explain the purpose of a *genogram*.

17. Explain the purpose of an *ecomap*.

Developmental assessment

18. Identify the seven family life cycle stages described by McGoldrick and Carter.
    a.
    b.
    c.
    d.
    e.
    f.
    g.

Copyright © 2019 Elsevier Canada, a division of Reed Elsevier Canada, Ltd.

19. Describe the two subcategories of *family functioning*.

 a. Instrumental functioning:

 ____

 ____

 b. Expressive functioning:

 ____

 ____

Family Intervention: The Calgary Family Intervention Model

20. Describe the ultimate goal of family intervention.

 ____

 ____

 ____

21. Name the three domains of family functioning that the Calgary Family Intervention Model (CFIM) focuses on promoting and improving.

 a. ______________________________

 b. ______________________________

 c. ______________________________

22. Describe the two types of interventive questions.

 a. *Linear questions*:

 ____

 ____

 b. *Circular questions*:

 ____

 ____

23. Describe the meaning of a *commendation* and why it is important for nurses to make commendations to families.

 ____

 ____

 ____

 ____

24. List five common family strengths.

 a. ______________________________

 b. ______________________________

 c. ______________________________

 d. ______________________________

 e. ______________________________

25. Family and patient needs for information may be elicited through direct questioning, but they are often ______________________________.

26. When you assume a humble, caring position instead of coming across as an authority on the subject, this attitude often decreases the patient's __________ and invites the family to listen without feeling ______________________________.

27. What is the purpose of validating emotional responses?

 ____

 ____

 ____

28. Describe an *illness narrative*.

 ____

 ____

 ____

 ____

29. You can enhance family functioning by encouraging and assisting family members to listen to each other's ______________ and ______________.

30. Describe the concept of *reciprocity*.

 ____

 ____

 ____

 ____

31. What are some of the benefits of *reciprocity*?

 ____

 ____

 ____

32. List nine community resources that may be beneficial to caregivers.

 a. ______________________________

 b. ______________________________

 c. ______________________________

 d. ______________________________

 e. ______________________________

 f. ______________________________

 g. ______________________________

 h. ______________________________

 i. ______________________________

Copyright © 2019 Elsevier Canada, a division of Reed Elsevier Canada, Ltd.

Interviewing the family

33. When interviewing the family, the nurse must display keen perceptual, conceptual, and executive skills. Describe each of these skills.

    a. Perceptual skills: ______

    b. Conceptual skills: ______

    c. Executive skills: ______

34. List five ways to engage in purposeful conversations with families.

    a. ______
    b. ______
    c. ______
    d. ______
    e. ______

REVIEW QUESTIONS

Select the appropriate answer, and cite the rationale for choosing that particular answer.

1. Family functioning can best be described as which of the following?
   a. The processes that a family uses to meet its goal
   b. The way the family members communicate with each other
   c. Interrelated with family structure
   d. Adaptive behaviours that foster health

Answer: ______ Rationale: ______

2. Family structure can best be described as which of the following?
   a. A basic pattern of predictable stages
   b. Flexible patterns that contribute to adequate functioning
   c. The pattern of relationships and ongoing membership
   d. A complex set of relationships

Answer: ______ Rationale: ______

3. "Skip-generation" families (grandparents caring for grandchildren), "nonfamilies" (adults living alone), and same-sex couples (with or without children) are considered which of the following?
   a. Diverse family forms
   b. Blended families
   c. Extended families
   d. Step-families

Answer: ______ Rationale: ______

4. In Canada, nurses could expect the following in respect to family forms and trends? *(Select all that apply.)*
   a. More one-person than couple households exist.
   b. Most children in lone-parent families live with a divorced or separated parent.
   c. More and more grandparents are caring for their grandchildren.
   d. There are increasing numbers of teenage mothers.

Answer: ______ Rationale: ______

5. When planning care for a patient and using the concept of family as patient, a nurse needs to do which of the following?
   a. Consider the developmental stage of the patient and not the family
   b. Realize that cultural background is an important variable when assessing the family
   c. Include only the patient and his or her significant other
   d. Understand that the patient's family will always be a help to the patient's health goals

Answer: ______ Rationale: ______

6. Interventions recommended by the CFIM include which of the following?
   a. Providing solutions for problems as they arise
   b. Validating emotional responses, encouraging illness narratives, and encouraging the patient to request help from his or her family
   c. Asking interventive questions, offering commendations, providing information, and encouraging respite
   d. Administering nursing care in a manner that provides an opportunity for change

Answer: ______ Rationale: ______

Copyright © 2019 Elsevier Canada, a division of Reed Elsevier Canada, Ltd.

20 Patient Education

PRELIMINARY READING

Chapter 20, pages 324–342

COMPREHENSIVE UNDERSTANDING

Patient education is one of the most important roles for nurses in any health care setting.

1. Identify three ways in which nurses are involved in the provision of information to patients.
   a. ____________________
   b. ____________________
   c. ____________________

2. Describe a *patient-centred* approach and the benefits of utilizing this approach.

____

Goals of Patient Education

3. Comprehensive patient education includes which three important goals?
   a. ____________________
   b. ____________________
   c. ____________________

4. Greater knowledge can result in __________. When patients become more __________, they are more likely to __________ and to __________.

5. Many patients seek __________ and __________ that will help them regain or maintain their levels of health.

6. The __________ is a vital part of a patient's return to health, and family members may need as much information as the patient.

7. Before you teach family members to assist the patient with health care management, it is important to assess the __________.

Teaching and Learning

8. Nurses have an __________ responsibility to teach their patients.

9. Effective teaching depends on __________.

Domains of Learning

10. List the three domains in which learning occurs.
    a. ____________________
    b. ____________________
    c. ____________________

Cognitive learning

11. *Cognitive learning* (Bloom, 1956) classifies cognitive behaviours in an ordered hierarchy. Summarize each one.
    a. Remembering:
    b. Understanding:
    c. Applying:
    d. Analyzing:
    e. Evaluating:
    f. Creating:

Copyright © 2019 Elsevier Canada, a division of Reed Elsevier Canada, Ltd.

12. Summarize the following hierarchy of *affective learning* behaviours.

    a. Receiving:

    b. Responding:

    c. Valuing:

    d. Organizing:

    e. Characterizing:

13. Summarize the following hierarchy of *psychomotor learning* behaviours.

    a. Perception:

    b. Set:

    c. Guided response:

    d. Mechanism:

    e. Complex overt response:

    f. Adaptation:

    g. Origination:

Basic Learning Principles

14. Factors in the physical environment where teaching takes place can make learning pleasant or difficult. List three factors to consider when selecting the learning setting.

    a. ______

    b. ______

    c. ______

15. Summarize how each of the following influences the ability to learn.

    a. Emotional capability:

    b. Intellectual capability:

    c. Physical capability:

    d. Developmental stage:

16. Everyone has different learning preferences and styles. You should ask patients their preferred method for learning. In a group, you should ______.

17. *Motivation* is defined as ______.

18. Briefly explain how the following can affect motivation.

    a. Social motives:

    b. Task mastery:

    c. Physical motives:

Copyright © 2019 Elsevier Canada, a division of Reed Elsevier Canada, Ltd.

19. Define *self-efficacy*.

____

____

20. The Transtheoretical Model of Change is utilized for smoking cessation. Identify the five stages in the model.

a. ____________________

b. ____________________

c. ____________________

d. ____________________

e. ____________________

Integrating the Nursing and Teaching Processes

21. Differentiate between the *nursing process* and the *teaching process*.

____

____

____

____

22. The teaching process requires ____________________ ____________________.

23. The nurse sets specific learning objectives and implements the teaching plan using teaching and learning principles to ensure ____________________ ____________________.

Assessment

24. The patient requires the nurse to assess the following factors. Summarize each one.

Learning needs:

a. ____________________

b. ____________________

c. ____________________

Ability to learn:

a. ____________________

b. ____________________

c. ____________________

d. ____________________

e. ____________________

Motivation to learn:

a. ____________________

b. ____________________

c. ____________________

d. ____________________

e. ____________________

f. ____________________

g. ____________________

h. ____________________

i. ____________________

Teaching environment:

a. ____________________

b. ____________________

c. ____________________

Resources for learning:

a. ____________________

b. ____________________

c. ____________________

d. ____________________

e. ____________________

Nursing Diagnosis

25. After assessing the patient's ability and need to learn, the nurse interprets data to form an ____________________ ____________________.

Planning

26. After determining the nursing diagnoses that identify a patient's learning needs, you develop a teaching plan, determine goals and expected outcomes, and involve the patient in a teaching method. Expected outcomes guide the ____________________ ____________________.

Developing learning objectives

27. A *learning objective* identifies the __________ of instruction and establishes ____________________ ____________________.

28. A learning objective includes the same criteria as goals or outcomes in a nursing care plan. These are as follows:

a. ____________________

b. ____________________

c. ____________________

d. ____________________

Copyright © 2019 Elsevier Canada, a division of Reed Elsevier Canada, Ltd.

29. The principles of teaching are techniques that incorporate the principles of learning. Explain the following principles.
   a. Setting priorities:
   b. Timing:
   c. Organizing teaching material:
   d. Maintaining attention and promoting participation:
   e. Building on existing knowledge:
   f. Selecting teaching methods:
   g. Selecting resources:
   h. Writing teaching plans:

Implementation

30. Briefly explain the following teaching approaches.
   a. Telling:
   b. Selling:
   c. Participating:
   d. Entrusting:
   e. Reinforcing:

31. Summarize the following instructional methods.
   a. One-on-one discussion:
   b. Group instruction:
   c. Preparatory instruction:
   d. Demonstrations:
   e. Analogies:
   f. Role playing:
   g. Simulation:

32. Identify some teaching strategies to be used with the following:
   a. Illiteracy and learning disability:
   b. Sensory alterations:
   c. Cultural diversity:
   d. Severe illness:

Copyright © 2019 Elsevier Canada, a division of Reed Elsevier Canada, Ltd.

Evaluation

33. Identify some evaluation measures.

____
____
____
____

34. List three areas to be included when documenting patient teaching.
   a. _______________
   b. _______________
   c. _______________

REVIEW QUESTIONS

Select the appropriate answer, and cite the rationale for choosing that particular answer.

1. A desire to learn is termed which of the following?
   a. Anxiety
   b. Motivation
   c. Compliance
   d. Adaptation

Answer: ___________ Rationale: ___________

2. Demonstration of the principles of body mechanics used when transferring patients from bed to chair would be classified under which domain of learning?
   a. Cognitive
   b. Social
   c. Psychomotor
   d. Affective

Answer: ___________ Rationale: ___________

3. Which of the following patients is most ready to begin a patient-teaching session?
   a. Ms. Benoit, who is unwilling to accept that her back injury may result in permanent paralysis
   b. Mr. Chang, a patient who recently received a diagnosis of diabetes, who is complaining that he was awake all night because of his noisy roommate
   c. Mrs. Ho, a patient with irritable bowel syndrome, who has just returned from a morning of testing in the gastroenterology laboratory
   d. Mr. Cinelli, a patient who had a heart attack 4 days ago and now seems somewhat anxious about how this will affect his future

Answer: ___________ Rationale: ___________

4. As a nurse, you work with pediatric patients who have diabetes. What is the youngest age group to which you can effectively teach psychomotor skills such as insulin administration?
   a. Toddler
   b. Adolescent
   c. School age
   d. Preschool

Answer: ___________ Rationale: ___________

5. Which of the following is an appropriately stated learning objective for Mr. Chang, who has just received a diagnosis of type 2 diabetes?
   a. Mr. Chang will be taught self-administration of insulin by May 2.
   b. Mr. Chang will perform blood glucose monitoring with the EZ-Check Monitor by the time of discharge.
   c. Mr. Chang will know the signs and symptoms of low blood sugar by May 5.
   d. Mr. Chang will understand diabetes.

Answer: ___________ Rationale: ___________

Copyright © 2019 Elsevier Canada, a division of Reed Elsevier Canada, Ltd.

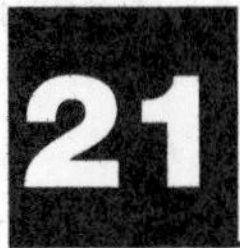

21 Developmental Theories

PRELIMINARY READING

Chapter 21, pages 343–359

COMPREHENSIVE UNDERSTANDING

Growth and Development

1. Define *growth.*

2. Define *development.*

Factors influencing growth and development

3. Identify the major factors influencing growth and development.
   a.
   b.
   c.

Traditions of Developmental Theories

4. List the five traditions of developmental theories.
   a.
   b.
   c.
   d.
   e.

5. Define *mechanisms of development.*

Organicism

6. Define *organicism.*

7. Briefly summarize Gesell's *theory of maturational development.*

8. Identify and describe the mechanisms of Gesell's theory.
   a.
   b.

9. Briefly describe Chess and Thomas's *theory of temperament development.*

10. Identify and describe the three categories of *temperament* in Chess and Thomas's theory.
    a.
    b.
    c.

11. Identify and describe the mechanisms of Chess and Thomas's theory.

Copyright © 2019 Elsevier Canada, a division of Reed Elsevier Canada, Ltd.

Cognitive developmental theories

12. Briefly summarize Piaget's *theory of cognitive development.*

13. Identify and describe the mechanisms of Piaget's theory.

    a.

    b.

14. Explain the four stages of Piaget's theory of cognitive development.

    a. Sensorimotor:

    b. Preoperational:

    c. Concrete operations:

    d. Formal operations:

15. Moral developmental theorists try to explain

16. Explain the three stages of Piaget's moral development theory.

    a. *Premoral stage*:

    b. *Conventional stage*:

    c. *Autonomous stage*:

17. Explain the six stages of Kohlberg's theory of moral development.

    a. Level I: Preconventional level

       Stage 1:

       Stage 2:

    b. Level II: Conventional level

       Stage 3:

       Stage 4:

    c. Level III: Postconventional level

       Stage 5:

       Stage 6:

18. Identify the limitations to Kohlberg's research.

19. Briefly explain Gilligan's argument against Kohlberg's theory.

Psychoanalytic and Psychosocial Tradition

20. What do theories in the psychoanalytic and psychosocial tradition describe?

21. Briefly summarize Freud's *psychoanalytic theory of personality development.*

Copyright © 2019 Elsevier Canada, a division of Reed Elsevier Canada, Ltd.

22. Identify and describe the mechanisms of Freud's theory.
    a. ______
    b. ______
    c. ______

23. Explain the five stages of Freud's theory.
    a. ______
    b. ______
    c. ______
    d. ______
    e. ______

24. Briefly summarize Erikson's *theory of psychosocial development*.

______

25. Identify and describe the mechanisms of Erikson's theory.
    a. ______
    b. ______

26. Explain the following eight stages of Erikson's theory.
    a. Trust versus mistrust:
    ______
    b. Autonomy versus shame and doubt:
    ______
    c. Initiative versus guilt:
    ______
    d. Industry versus inferiority:
    ______
    e. Identity versus role confusion:
    ______
    f. Intimacy versus isolation:
    ______
    g. Generativity versus self-absorption and stagnation:
    ______
    h. Integrity versus despair:
    ______

27. Define *attachment* according to Crittenden's dynamic maturational model.

______

28. Briefly summarize Havighurst's theory of development.

______

29. Identify a limitation to Havighurst's theory.

______

30. Havighurst defined a series of essential tasks that arise from predictable and external pressures. These pressures include ______, ______, and ______.

Mechanistic Tradition

31. Briefly explain the *mechanistic tradition*.

______

Contextualism

32. Developmental theories within the *contextual tradition* focus on ______.

33. Briefly summarize Bronfenbrenner's *bioecologic theory of development*.

______

Copyright © 2019 Elsevier Canada, a division of Reed Elsevier Canada, Ltd.

34. Explain the four "layers" of environment in Bronfenbrenner's theory.
    a. ____________________
    b. ____________________
    c. ____________________
    d. ____________________

35. Identify and describe the mechanisms of Bronfenbrenner's theory.

____

____

Dialecticism

36. Briefly explain the *dialectic tradition.*

____

____

____

37. Briefly summarize Keating and Hertzman's *population health approach.*

____

____

____

38. Identify and describe the mechanisms of Keating and Hertzman's theory.
    a. ____________________
    b. ____________________
    c. ____________________

39. Briefly describe the *resilience* approach to development.

____

____

____

40. Identify and describe the mechanisms of Resilience theory.
    a. ____________________
    b. ____________________

Developmental Theories and Nursing

41. A clear understanding of patterns of growth and development and of the contexts within which they occur assist you in ____________________ and ____________________ and in ____________________. You need to consider an individual's development within the ____________ of his or her families, social relationships, communities, and the larger society.

REVIEW QUESTIONS

Select the appropriate answer, and cite the rationale for choosing that particular answer.

1. According to Piaget, the school-aged child is in the third stage of cognitive development, which is characterized by which of the following?
   a. Conventional thought
   b. Concrete operations
   c. Identity versus role diffusion
   d. Postconventional thought

Answer:____________ Rationale:____________

____

____

2. According to Bronfenbrenner's developmental theory, the individual and his or her environment are seen as mutually influential. Development of a national child care policy is an example of an intervention at which level?
   a. Microsystem
   b. Mesosystem
   c. Exosystem
   d. Macrosystem

Answer:____________ Rationale:____________

____

____

3. According to Erikson's developmental theory, the primary developmental task of the middle adult years is which of the following?
   a. Achieve generativity
   b. Achieve intimacy
   c. Establish a set of personal values
   d. Establish a sense of personal identity

Answer:____________ Rationale:____________

____

____

4. Which of the following behaviours is most characteristic of the concrete operations stage of cognitive development?
   a. There is progression from reflex activity to imitative behaviour.
   b. There is inability to put oneself in another's place.
   c. Thought processes become increasingly logical and coherent.
   d. The ability to think in abstract terms and draw logical conclusions develops.

Answer:____________ Rationale:____________

____

____

Copyright © 2019 Elsevier Canada, a division of Reed Elsevier Canada, Ltd.

5. According to Kohlberg, children develop moral reasoning as they mature. Which of the following is most characteristic of a preschooler's stage of moral development?
   a. It is important to obey the rules of correct behaviour.
   b. Showing respect for authority is important behaviour.
   c. Behaviour that pleases others is considered good.
   d. Actions are determined as good or bad in terms of their consequences.

Answer:_______________ Rationale:_______________

____

____

Copyright © 2019 Elsevier Canada, a division of Reed Elsevier Canada, Ltd.

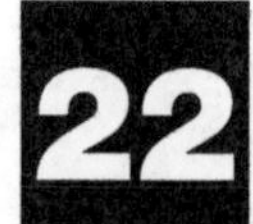

22 Conception Through Adolescence

PRELIMINARY READING

Chapter 22, pages 360–396

COMPREHENSIVE UNDERSTANDING

Human growth and development are continuous, intricate, and complex processes that are often divided into stages organized by age groups.

Selecting a Developmental Framework for Nursing

1. When utilizing a developmental approach, care is ____, ________________, and ____________________.

Conception

2. Define the following terms or events.

   a. *Nagele's rule*:

   b. *Fertilization*:

   c. *Zygote*:

   d. *Morula*:

   e. *Blastocyst*:

   f. *Embryo*:

   g. *Placenta*:

   h. *Implantation*:

3. Explain the development process and health concerns for the following trimesters.

   a. First trimester

   Physical changes:

   Health concerns:

   Teratogens:

   b. Second trimester

   Physical changes:

   Health concerns:

   c. Third trimester

   Physical changes:

   Health concerns:

Transition from Intrauterine to Extrauterine Life

4. ____________, ____________, and ____________ changes all contribute to the infant's adaptation to neonatal life.

Copyright © 2019 Elsevier Canada, a division of Reed Elsevier Canada, Ltd.

5. List the five physiologic parameters evaluated through the *Apgar* assessment.
   a. ___
   b. ___
   c. ___
   d. ___
   e. ___
6. What time period after birth is optimal for parent–neonate interaction to begin?

___

7. Define *bonding*.

___

___

8. Briefly explain the three most important physical needs of the newborn in each category.
   a. Airway:
   ___
   ___
   b. Temperature:
   ___
   ___
   c. Prevention of infection:
   ___
   ___

Newborn

9. The neonatal period is defined as ___

___.

10. Identify the normal characteristics of the newborn.
   a. Height: ___
   b. Weight: ___
   c. Head circumference: ___
   d. Vital signs: ___
   ___
   ___
   e. Physical characteristics: ___
   ___
   f. Neurologic function: ___
   ___
   g. Behavioural characteristics: ___
   ___

11. Identify the sensory functions that contribute to cognitive development in the newborn.

___

___

12. Explain the interactions that foster deep attachment between the infant and the parents.

___

___

13. Define *hyperbilirubinemia*.

___

___

14. Screening for inborn errors of metabolism applies to

___

___.

15. Circumcision is a common and controversial procedure. Identify the risks of this procedure.

___

___

Infant

16. Infancy is the period from ___ to ___.
17. Summarize the normal characteristics of the infant.
   a. Physical growth:
   ___
   ___
   b. Vital signs:
   ___
   ___
18. Summarize the cognitive development of an infant.

___

___

___

19. Define *play*.

___

___

20. Identify activities that are appropriate for the infant stage of development.

___

___

___

Copyright © 2019 Elsevier Canada, a division of Reed Elsevier Canada, Ltd.

21. Identify the common types of injury in infants and possible prevention strategies.

22. Child maltreatment includes ________________.

23. Identify the feeding alternatives for an infant.

24. Identify some supplementation needs of an infant.

25. Briefly explain health concerns in infants related to the following:

a. Dentition:

b. Immunizations:

c. Sleep:

Toddler

26. Toddlerhood ranges from __________ to __________.

27. Summarize the normal characteristics of a toddler.

a. Self-care activities:

b. Motor skills:

c. Vital signs:

d. Weight:

e. Height:

28. Summarize Piaget's *preoperational* thought stage.

29. Describe the language ability of toddlers.

30. According to Erikson, what psychosocial development is considered appropriate in toddlers?

31. Describe some developmental abilities that increase the risk of injury for toddlers.

32. What are the seven main areas of concern in injury prevention for toddlers?

a.

b.

c.

d.

e.

f.

g.

33. Briefly explain the nutrition requirements for toddlers.

Copyright © 2019 Elsevier Canada, a division of Reed Elsevier Canada, Ltd.

Preschooler

34. The preschool period refers to ______________________________.

35. Summarize the normal characteristics of the preschooler.

    a. Vital signs: ______________________________

    b. Weight: ______________________________

    c. Height: ______________________________

    d. Coordination: ______________________________

Preschoolers continue to master the preoperational stage of cognition.

36. The first phase of this period (2 to 4 years) is characterized by ______________________________.

37. Define *artificialism.* ______________________________

38. Define *animism.* ______________________________

39. Define *immanent justice.* ______________________________

40. Summarize the intuitive phase of preoperational thought (4 years). ______________________________

41. The greatest fear of preschoolers is ______________________________.

42. Summarize the moral development of preschoolers. ______________________________

43. Describe the language ability of preschoolers. ______________________________

44. Identify some dependent behaviours that preschoolers may revert to during stress or illness. ______________________________

45. Summarize the pattern of play for the preschooler. ______________________________

46. Guidelines for injury prevention in the toddler also apply to the preschooler. __________ and __________ remain the leading causes of injury for this age group.

47. Explain health concerns related to the following for preschoolers.

    a. Nutrition: ______________________________

    b. Sleep: ______________________________

    c. Vision: ______________________________

School-Aged Children and Adolescents

48. The school-age years range from __________ to _______ years of age.

49. __________, which occurs at about 12 years of age, signals the end of middle childhood.

Copyright © 2019 Elsevier Canada, a division of Reed Elsevier Canada, Ltd.

50. Summarize the normal characteristics of the school-aged child.

    a. Weight:

    ____

    ____

    b. Height:

    ____

    ____

    c. Cardiovascular functioning:

    ____

    ____

    d. Neuromuscular functioning:

    ____

    ____

    e. Skeletal growth:

    ____

    ____

51. Define the cognitive skills that are developing in the school-aged group.

    ____

    ____

    ____

    ____

52. Describe language development during middle childhood.

    ____

    ____

    ____

    ____

53. The developmental task for school-aged children is __________ versus __________.

54. Summarize psychosocial development in school-aged children in relation to the following:

    a. Moral development:

    ____

    ____

    b. Peer relationships:

    ____

    ____

    c. Sexual identity:

    ____

    ____

55. ______________________________ and ______________________________ are the leading causes of death or injury.

56. Identify the specific health concerns of children living in poverty.

    ____

    ____

    ____

57. Identify five critical functions of a school-based health promotion program.

    a. ______________________________
    b. ______________________________
    c. ______________________________
    d. ______________________________
    e. ______________________________

58. Identify at least five health promotion activities that are appropriate for the school-aged child.

    a. ______________________________
    b. ______________________________
    c. ______________________________
    d. ______________________________
    e. ______________________________

59. Identify the nutritional requirements for the school-aged child.

    ____

    ____

    ____

    ____

Adolescent

60. Adolescence is the period of development ______________________________.

61. Define *puberty* and explain the changes that occur at this time.

    ____

    ____

    ____

62. List the four major physical changes associated with sexual maturation.

    a. ______________________________
    b. ______________________________
    c. ______________________________
    d. ______________________________

Copyright © 2019 Elsevier Canada, a division of Reed Elsevier Canada, Ltd.

63. The hormones responsible for the development of secondary sex characteristics are __________ and __________.

64. Summarize the weight and skeletal changes that occur during adolescence.

65. Explain the effects of physical changes on peer interactions among adolescents.

66. Changes that occur within the mind and the widening social environment of the adolescent result in __________ __________, the highest level of intellectual development.

67. Briefly explain the cognitive abilities of adolescents.

68. Describe the language skills of the adolescent.

69. The search for __________ is the major task of adolescent psychosocial development.

70. Explain identity (or role) confusion (Erikson).

71. Behaviours in adolescents that indicate a lack of resolution are __________ and __________.

72. Explain the following components of total identity.

a. Gender identity: __________

b. Group identity: __________

c. Family identity: __________

d. Vocational identity: __________

e. Moral identity: __________

f. Health identity: __________

73. Identify the leading cause of death and its sources among adolescents.

74. Suicide is the second leading cause of death among adolescents. List the six warning signs of suicide for this group.

a.

b.

c.

d.

e.

f.

75. Substance abuse is a major concern. Adolescents most at risk are those coming from __________ __________.

76. Eating disorders are on the rise among adolescents. Define the following eating disorders.

a. Anorexia nervosa:

b. Bulimia nervosa:

77. __________, __________, and __________ expectations contribute to early heterosexual and homosexual relations among adolescents.

78. Briefly explain the two prominent consequences of adolescent sexual activity.

a. Sexually transmitted infections (STIs):

Copyright © 2019 Elsevier Canada, a division of Reed Elsevier Canada, Ltd.

b. Pregnancy:

79. Identify health promotion interventions for the adolescent in regard to the following:

a. Unintentional injuries:

b. Firearm use and violence:

c. Substance use:

d. Suicide:

e. Sexual activity:

80. Identify the health concerns of the following:

a. Adolescents in rural communities:

b. Minority adolescents:

c. Indigenous adolescents:

d. Lesbian, gay, bisexual, and transgender adolescents:

REVIEW QUESTIONS

Select the appropriate answer, and cite the rationale for choosing that particular answer.

1. Which statement about human growth and development is accurate?
   a. Growth and development processes are unpredictable.
   b. Growth and development begin with birth and end after adolescence.
   c. All individuals progress through the same phases of growth and development.
   d. All individuals accomplish developmental tasks at the same pace.

Answer:__________ Rationale:__________

2. The mother of a 2-year-old expresses concern that her son's appetite has diminished and that he seems to prefer milk to solid foods. Which response reflects your knowledge of the principles of communication and nutrition?
   a. "Oh, I wouldn't be too worried; children tend to eat when they're hungry. I just wouldn't give him dessert unless he eats his meal."
   b. "That is not uncommon in toddlers. You might consider increasing his milk to 2 L per day to be sure he gets enough nutrients."
   c. "Have you considered feeding him when he doesn't seem interested in feeding himself?"
   d. "A toddler's rate of growth normally slows down. It's common to see a toddler's appetite diminish in response to decreased calorie needs."

Answer:__________ Rationale:__________

3. Which neonatal assessment finding would be considered abnormal?
   a. Cyanosis of the hands and feet during activity
   b. Palpable anterior and posterior fontanels
   c. Soft, protuberant abdomen
   d. Absence of the rooting, grasping, and sucking reflexes

Answer:__________ Rationale:__________

4. To stimulate cognitive and psychosocial development of the toddler, it is important for parents to do which of the following?
   a. Set firm and consistent limits
   b. Foster sharing of toys with playmates and siblings
   c. Provide clarification about what is right and wrong
   d. Allow complete freedom for exploration of the environment

Answer:__________ Rationale:__________

Copyright © 2019 Elsevier Canada, a division of Reed Elsevier Canada, Ltd.

5. Which of the following statements is true of the developmental behaviours of school-aged children?
   a. Formal and informal peer group membership is the key to forming self-esteem.
   b. Fears centre on the loss of self-control.
   c. Positive feedback from parents and teachers is crucial to development.
   d. A full range of defence mechanisms is used, including rationalization and intellectualization.

Answer:__________ Rationale:__________

6. Adolescents have mastered age-appropriate sexuality when they feel comfortable with which of the following? *(Select all that apply.)*
   a. Sexual behaviours
   b. Sexual choices
   c. Sexual relationships
   d. All of these

Answer:__________ Rationale:__________

Copyright © 2019 Elsevier Canada, a division of Reed Elsevier Canada, Ltd.

23 Young to Middle Adulthood

PRELIMINARY READING

Chapter 23, pages 397–410

COMPREHENSIVE UNDERSTANDING

1. Young adulthood is the period from ________ ________ to ________.
2. Individuals in young adulthood ________, ________, and ________ ________.
3. Middle age occurs from ________ to ________.
4. Middle-aged adults become aware of changes in ________ and ________ abilities. This is a time when individuals may reassess ________.

Young Adulthood

5. The young adult has completed physical growth by the age of 20. List the characteristics of young adults.
   a. ________
   b. ________
   c. ________
   d. ________
6. Identify the main components of a personal lifestyle assessment of a young adult.
   ____
   ____
   ____
7. Formal and informal education, life experiences, and work opportunities increase the young adult's ________ and ________ skills.
8. Choosing an occupation is a ________ of young adults and involves knowing their ________, ________, and ________.
9. Explain the teach-back technique that is used to increase health literacy.
   ____
   ____
10. The emotional health of the young adult is related to the individual's ability to address and resolve personal and social tasks. Explain the patterns of change that are common in the following age groups.
    a. 23 to 28 years:
    ____
    ____
    b. 29 to 34 years:
    ____
    ____
11. ________ and ________ issues influence an adult's life and can pose challenges for nursing care.
12. For young men and women, successful employment ensures ________ and promotes ________, ________, ________, and ________.
13. In two-career partnerships, the ________ ________ may outweigh ________ ________.
14. Describe trends in families and living arrangements in Canada.
    ____
    ____
15. Close friends and associates of the single young adult may also be viewed as the individual's ________.
16. Identify five tasks to be completed by a couple before marriage.
    a. ________
    b. ________
    c. ________
    d. ________
    e. ________

Copyright © 2019 Elsevier Canada, a division of Reed Elsevier Canada, Ltd.

17. What knowledge do nurses need to support a transmasculine person who is involved in infant feeding?

___

___

18. During a psychologic assessment of young adults, the nurse can assess for ___ of emotional health that indicate successful maturation in this developmental stage.

19. Briefly explain the risk factors for young adults in regard to the following:

a. Lifestyle:

___

___

b. Family history:

___

___

c. Accidental death and injury:

___

___

d. Substance abuse:

___

___

e. Unplanned pregnancies:

___

___

f. Sexually transmitted infections (STIs):

___

___

g. Environmental and occupational factors:

___

___

20. Give examples of nursing assessment and interventions for young adults related to the following areas of health.

a. Infertility:

___

___

b. Exercise:

___

___

c. Routine health screening:

___

___

21. The psychosocial concerns of the young adult are often related to stress. Briefly explain each of the following sources of stress.

a. Job stress:

___

___

b. Family stress:

___

___

22. Explain the health practices that you would discuss with a woman anticipating pregnancy.

___

___

___

___

___

___

23. *Prenatal care* is

___.

24. Explain the implications for nursing associated with the following psychosocial changes that occur during pregnancy.

a. Body image:

___

___

b. Role changes:

___

___

c. Sexuality:

___

___

d. Coping mechanisms:

___

___

e. Stresses during puerperium:

___

___

Copyright © 2019 Elsevier Canada, a division of Reed Elsevier Canada, Ltd.

f. Postpartum blues and depression:

25. Provide examples of when acute care might be required for young adults.

26. Describe the effect of chronic illness and disability on the young adult.

Middle Adulthood

27. Briefly explain the characteristics of the middle adult years.

28. Briefly explain the major physiologic changes that occur between 40 and 65 years of age.

29. Define *menopause*.

30. Define *sandwich generation*.

31. Summarize the psychosocial development of the middle-aged adult in the following areas.

a. Career transition:

b. Sexuality:

c. Family types:

d. Singlehood:

e. Marital changes:

f. Family transitions:

g. Care of aging parents:

32. Briefly explain each of the following physiologic concerns for the middle-aged adult and suggest appropriate nursing assessment and interventions.

a. Stress and stress reduction:

b. Obesity:

33. List some positive health habits that support health for the middle-aged adult.

34. ____________ and ____________ are often directed at improving health habits.

35. Identify three external barriers to health literacy.

a. ____________

b. ____________

c. ____________

36. Identify four internal barriers to health literacy.

a. ____________

b. ____________

c. ____________

d. ____________

Copyright © 2019 Elsevier Canada, a division of Reed Elsevier Canada, Ltd.

37. Summarize two psychosocial concerns of the middle-aged adult, and provide the appropriate nursing assessment and interventions.

a. Anxiety:

____

____

____

b. Depression:

____

____

____

38. Primary health care programs for young and middle adults are designed to ______________, ______________, and ______________.

39. How do injuries and acute illnesses differ in middle childhood from those experienced in young adulthood?

____

____

____

40. Identify some chronic illnesses or issues that occur in middle adulthood.

____

____

____

REVIEW QUESTIONS

Select the appropriate answer, and cite the rationale for choosing that particular answer.

1. The leading cause of injury and death in the young adult population is which of the following?
   a. Sexually transmitted infection
   b. Accidents
   c. Cardiovascular disease
   d. Substance abuse

Answer: ______________ Rationale: ______________

____

____

2. Psychosocial changes of pregnancy commonly involve all of these areas, *except* which of the following?
   a. Altered body image
   b. Reduced stress
   c. Role changes
   d. Sexuality

Answer: ______________ Rationale: ______________

____

____

3. Which physiologic change would be a normal assessment finding in a middle-aged adult? *(Select all that apply.)*
   a. Increased breast size
   b. Abdominal tenderness
   c. Decreased skin turgor
   d. Increased thoracic diameter
   e. Reduced auditory acuity

Answer: ______________ Rationale: ______________

____

____

4. Which of the following is most likely to affect the overall level of health of a patient in middle adulthood?
   a. Stress due to life changes
   b. Decreased visual acuity
   c. Declining sexual interest
   d. Onset of menopause

Answer: ______________ Rationale: ______________

____

____

5. In planning patient education for Fran Higuchi, a 45-year-old woman who had an ovarian cyst removed, which of the following facts is true about the sexuality of the middle-aged adult?
   a. Menstruation ceases after menopause.
   b. Estrogen is produced after menopause.
   c. Middle-aged men are unable to produce fertile sperm.
   d. With removal of an ovarian cyst, pregnancy cannot occur.

Answer: ______________ Rationale: ______________

____

____

Copyright © 2019 Elsevier Canada, a division of Reed Elsevier Canada, Ltd.

24 Older Persons

PRELIMINARY READING

Chapter 24, pages 411–431

COMPREHENSIVE UNDERSTANDING

1. Briefly summarize demographic trends of older Canadians.

___
___
___
___

Variability Among Older Persons

2. Briefly explain changes of the older person.

   a. Physiologic:

   ___
   ___

   b. Cognitive and psychosocial:

   ___
   ___
   ___
   ___

Myths and Stereotypes

3. Identify at least five myths or stereotypes regarding the older person.

   a. ___
   b. ___
   c. ___
   d. ___
   e. ___
   ___

4. Define *ageism*.

___
___

Nurses' Attitudes Toward Older Persons

5. The attitude of the nurse toward older persons comes in part from ___, ___, ___, and ___.

6. List the seven developmental tasks of the older person.

   a. ___
   b. ___
   c. ___
   d. ___
   e. ___
   f. ___
   g. ___

Aging Well and Quality of Life

7. Older persons are considered to be ___ when they are ___
___.

Community-Based and Institutional Health Care Services

8. Briefly describe the following health services that are used by older persons.

   a. Long-term care facilities:

   ___
   ___

   b. Assisted-living facilities:

   ___
   ___

   c. Personal care homes:

   ___
   ___

9. Describe the services provided to older persons by each of the following:

   a. Senior centres: ___
   ___

   b. Companions and friendly visitors: ___
   ___

   c. Home-delivered meals: ___
   ___

Copyright © 2019 Elsevier Canada, a division of Reed Elsevier Canada, Ltd.

d. Telephone reassurance: ____________________

e. Personal emergency response systems: ____________________

f. Energy assistance programs: ____________________

Assessing the Needs of Older Persons

10. Nurses need to take into account five key points to ensure an age-specific approach.
    a. ____________________
    b. ____________________
    c. ____________________
    d. ____________________
    e. ____________________

11. Explain why an assessment with an older person may require more time than with a younger adult.

12. Identify the physiologic changes that occur in the older person with regard to the following systems.
    a. Integumentary system:
    b. Respiratory system:
    c. Cardiovascular system:
    d. Gastrointestinal system:
    e. Musculoskeletal system:
    f. Neurologic system:
    g. Sensory system:
    h. Genitourinary system:
    i. Reproductive system:
    j. Endocrine system:
    k. Immune system:

Functional changes

13. *Functional status* in older persons ordinarily refers to the capacity and safe performance of activities of daily living, and it is a sensitive indicator of health or illness in older persons. Factors that promote the highest level of functioning in all areas include:
    a. ____________________
    b. ____________________
    c. ____________________
    d. ____________________
    e. ____________________
    f. ____________________

14. Define the following terms.
    a. *Delirium*:
    b. *Dementia*:
    c. *Depression*:

Copyright © 2019 Elsevier Canada, a division of Reed Elsevier Canada, Ltd.

15. Identify the characteristic progressive symptoms of *Alzheimer's disease.*
    a. ______
    b. ______
    c. ______
    d. ______

16. Identify four nonpharmacologic measures that a nurse could utilize with persons who have dementia, rather than using restraints.
    a. ______
    b. ______
    c. ______
    d. ______

17. Briefly explain some of the reasons older persons experience social isolation.

______

18. Elder abuse is the mistreatment of an older person by other people who are in a position of trust or power or who are responsible for the person's care. List the six types of abuse, and discuss the role of the nurse.
    a. ______
    b. ______
    c. ______
    d. ______
    e. ______
    f. ______

19. Briefly describe the sexual changes that occur in the older person.

______

20. List four factors to assess when assisting older persons with housing needs.
    a. ______
    b. ______
    c. ______
    d. ______

21. Define *age-friendly community.*

______

Addressing the Health Concerns of Older Persons

22. The two most common causes of death in the older person are ______ and ______.

23. Summarize the physiologic health concerns related to each of the following:
    a. Cancer: ______
    b. Heart disease: ______
    c. Smoking: ______
    d. Alcohol abuse: ______
    e. Nutrition: ______
    f. Oral health: ______
    g. Exercise: ______
    h. Arthritis: ______
    i. Falls: ______
    j. Sensory impairments: ______
    k. Pain: ______

Copyright © 2019 Elsevier Canada, a division of Reed Elsevier Canada, Ltd.

l. Medication use:

Health promotion and maintenance: psychosocial health concerns

24. Briefly describe the interventions used to maintain the psychosocial health of the older adult.

  a. Therapeutic communication:

  b. Touch:

  c. Cognitive stimulation:

  d. Reminiscence:

  e. Body-image interventions:

Older Persons and the Acute Care Setting

25. Explain why the older person is at risk for each of the following:

  a. Delirium:

  b. Dehydration:

  c. Malnutrition:

  d. Nosocomial infections:

  e. Urinary incontinence:

  f. Falls:

Older Persons and Restorative Care

26. Summarize the two types of ongoing care for the older person and identify the focus of each.

Older Persons and Palliative Care

27. Describe the purpose of *palliative care.*

REVIEW QUESTIONS

Select the appropriate answer and cite the rationale for choosing that particular answer.

1. Which statement about older persons is accurate?
   a. Older persons are institutionalized.
   b. Most older persons live on a fixed income.
   c. Most older persons cannot learn to care for themselves.
   d. Most older persons have no sexual desire.

Answer:________ Rationale:________

2. Which statement describing *delirium* is correct?
   a. Persons with delirium may experience hallucinations.
   b. The onset of delirium is slow and insidious.
   c. Symptoms of delirium are stable and unchanging.
   d. Symptoms of delirium are irreversible.

Answer:________ Rationale:________

Copyright © 2019 Elsevier Canada, a division of Reed Elsevier Canada, Ltd.

3. Which of the following actions would be helpful when communicating with an older person with a sensory impairment? *(Select all that apply.)*
   a. Use a loud voice
   b. Use a high-pitched voice
   c. Speak slowly
   d. Avoid touching

Answer:______________ Rationale:______________

____

____

4. Which of the following contributes to polypharmacy?
   a. Substance abuse in older persons
   b. Multiple, concurrent health disorders
   c. Adverse side effects from inappropriate prescribing of sedatives
   d. Marketing of new medications by drug companies

Answer:______________ Rationale:______________

____

____

5. Which of the following describes palliative care?
   a. It is available only at the end of life.
   b. Its primary focus is cure of underlying disorders.
   c. It is applicable only to older persons.
   d. It meets a full range of needs early on in chronic disease and at end of life.
   e. It is an integrated approach that involves patients, families, and professionals in management of symptoms.

Answer:______________ Rationale:______________

____

____

Copyright © 2019 Elsevier Canada, a division of Reed Elsevier Canada, Ltd.

25 The Experience of Loss, Death, and Grief

PRELIMINARY READING

Chapter 25, pages 432–456

COMPREHENSIVE UNDERSTANDING

Loss and grief are experiences that affect not only patients and their families but the nurses who care for them as well.

Scientific Knowledge Base

1. Give an example of the five categories of loss.

   a. Necessary loss:

   b. Actual loss:

   c. Perceived loss:

   d. Maturational loss:

   e. Situational loss:

2. Describe the following terms.

   a. *Grief*:

   b. *Bereavement*:

3. List the phases of the grieving process proposed by each of the theorists listed.

   a. Kübler-Ross's Stages of Grief:

   i.
   ii.
   iii.
   iv.
   v.

   b. Bowlby's Phases of Mourning:

   i.
   ii.
   iii.
   iv.

   c. Worden's Four Tasks of Mourning:

   i.
   ii.
   iii.
   iv.

4. Briefly describe the following types of grief.

   a. Normal grief:

   b. Anticipatory grief:

   c. Complicated grief:

Copyright © 2019 Elsevier Canada, a division of Reed Elsevier Canada, Ltd.

d. Disenfranchised grief:

____

____

Nursing Knowledge Base

5. Briefly explain the factors that influence loss and grief.

a. Human development:

____

____

____

b. Psychosocial perspectives:

____

____

____

c. Socioeconomic status:

____

____

____

d. Personal relationships:

____

____

____

e. Nature of the loss:

____

____

____

f. Culture and ethnicity:

____

____

____

g. Spiritual beliefs:

____

____

____

6. Explain how the mechanism of *hope* is used to cope with grief and loss.

____

____

____

____

Critical Thinking

7. Knowledge of the stages of grief enables you to ____________________ and to understand ____________________. Through identification of the stages of grief, you are able to ____________________.

The Nursing Process and Grief

Assessment

8. Identify some symptoms of normal grief feelings.

____

____

____

____

9. List four of the factors that affect grief.

____

____

____

____

10. Briefly explain *end-of-life decisions*.

____

____

____

____

11. Explain how nurses are involved in MAID.

____

____

____

____

12. It is normal to have ____________________ and ____________________ about illness and death. It is inappropriate to emphasize ____________________.

Nursing Diagnosis

13. List four possible nursing diagnoses for patients or families experiencing grief.

a. ____________________

b. ____________________

c. ____________________

d. ____________________

Copyright © 2019 Elsevier Canada, a division of Reed Elsevier Canada, Ltd.

Planning

14. List three expected outcomes appropriate for a patient dealing with loss.
    a. ______
    b. ______
    c. ______

15. Briefly explain how to prioritize the needs of the grieving patient.

______

Implementation

16. Describe five therapeutic communication strategies you can use to help patients discuss and work through their loss.
    a. ______
    b. ______
    c. ______
    d. ______
    e. ______

17. Give an example of a nursing strategy to promote hope for each dimension.
    a. Affective dimension:
    b. Cognitive dimension:
    c. Behavioural dimension:
    d. Affiliative dimension:
    e. Temporal dimension:
    f. Contextual dimension:

18. Identify the nursing strategies to facilitate mourning for the patient and family.
    a. ______
    b. ______
    c. ______
    d. ______
    e. ______
    f. ______
    g. ______

19. According to the World Health Organization, when health care providers deliver palliative care, they do the following:
    a. ______
    b. ______
    c. ______
    d. ______
    e. ______
    f. ______
    g. ______

20. Give examples of how the following contribute to comfort for the dying patient.
    a. Symptom control:
    b. Maintaining dignity and self-esteem:
    c. Preventing abandonment and isolation:
    d. Providing a comfortable and peaceful environment:

21. Describe seven teaching strategies to prepare the dying patient's family.
    a. ______
    b. ______
    c. ______
    d. ______
    e. ______
    f. ______
    g. ______

Copyright © 2019 Elsevier Canada, a division of Reed Elsevier Canada, Ltd.

22. Identify the components of *hospice* care.
    a. ______
    b. ______
    c. ______
    d. ______
    e. ______
    f. ______
    g. ______
    h. ______

23. Explain how you can support the family through the organ and tissue request or donation process.

______

24. The family becomes ______ when the ______ has occurred, and the shift ______ to the living family.

Evaluation

25. The success of evaluation depends partially on ______.

REVIEW QUESTIONS

Select the appropriate answer, and cite the rationale for choosing that particular answer.

1. Which statement about loss is accurate?
   a. Loss is experienced only when something valued is actually absent.
   b. The more an individual has invested in what is lost, the less the feeling of loss.
   c. Loss may be maturational, situational, or both.
   d. The degree of stress experienced is unrelated to the type of loss.

Answer: ______ Rationale: ______

2. A hospice program emphasizes which of the following?
   a. Curative treatment and alleviation of symptoms
   b. Palliative treatment and control of symptoms
   c. Hospital-based care
   d. Prolongation of life

Answer: ______ Rationale: ______

3. Trying uncertain forms of complementary therapy is a behaviour that is characteristic of which stage of dying?
   a. Anger
   b. Depression
   c. Bargaining
   d. Acceptance

Answer: ______ Rationale: ______

4. All of the following are crucial needs of the dying patient *except* which one?
   a. Control of pain
   b. Preservation of dignity and self-worth
   c. Love and belonging
   d. Freedom from decision making

Answer: ______ Rationale: ______

5. A patient is experiencing great anxiety about air hunger. Which of the following interventions may assist to relieve the air hunger? *(Select all that apply.)*
   a. Position patient in semi-Fowler's position.
   b. Administer diuretics if ordered.
   c. Collaborate with patient and family regarding interventions.
   d. Administer morphine.
   e. Change oxygen devices.

Answer: ______ Rationale: ______

Copyright © 2019 Elsevier Canada, a division of Reed Elsevier Canada, Ltd.

26 Self-Concept

PRELIMINARY READING

Chapter 26, pages 457–475

COMPREHENSIVE UNDERSTANDING

1. *Self-concept* is often considered the ____________ ______________________, while *self-esteem* refers to the extent to which ______________ ______________________.

Scientific Knowledge Base

2. Explain how the level of self-esteem varies across the lifespan.

Nursing Knowledge Base

3. Each stage of development has specific activities that assist the patient in developing a positive self-concept. Identify some activities for each stage.

   a. 0 to 1 year:

   b. 1 to 3 years:

   c. 3 to 6 years:

   d. 6 to 12 years:

   e. 12 to 20 years:

   f. Mid-20s to mid-40s:

   g. Mid-40s to mid-60s:

   h. Late 60s on:

4. Self-concept is a dynamic perception that is based on the following:

   a. ______
   b. ______
   c. ______
   d. ______
   e. ______
   f. ______
   g. ______
   h. ______
   i. ______
   j. ______
   k. ______
   l. ______
   m. ______

5. Briefly explain the four significant components of self-concept.

   a. *Identity*:

Copyright © 2019 Elsevier Canada, a division of Reed Elsevier Canada, Ltd.

b. *Body image*:

c. *Self-esteem*:

d. *Role performance*:

6. List the processes through which an individual learns appropriate behaviours.

a.
b.
c.
d.
e.

7. A self-concept stressor is any ______________.

8. Define *identity confusion.*

9. Changes in the appearance, structure, or function of a body part will require a change in body image. Identify at least five stressors that affect body image.

a.
b.
c.
d.
e.

10. Explain how transitions within one's roles may lead to the following:

a. *Role conflict*:

b. *Role ambiguity*:

c. *Role strain*:

d. *Role overload*:

The Family's Effect on Development of Self-Concept

11. Explain how the attachment of children to their caregivers influences the development of self-concept.

12. List five areas you, as nurse, must clarify and assess about yourself to promote a positive self-concept in clients.

a.
b.
c.
d.
e.

Critical Thinking

13. ______________ influences a person's response to illness.

Self-Concept and the Nursing Process

Assessment

14. In assessing self-concept, you should focus on each component related to self-concept and observe for behaviours suggestive of ______________, actual and potential self-concept ______________, and ______________ patterns.

15. The nursing assessment should include consideration of previous coping behaviours: the ______________, ______________, and ______________ of the stressors; and the client's ______________ and ______________ resources.

Copyright © 2019 Elsevier Canada, a division of Reed Elsevier Canada, Ltd.

16. Asking the client how he or she believes interventions will make a difference in the problem can provide useful information regarding the client's expectations and can provide an opportunity to discuss the client's goals. Give an example.

____

____

Nursing Diagnosis

17. Provide two examples of diagnoses related to self-concept.

____

____

Planning

18. Before involving the family, you need to consider the ______________________ and ______________ ______________________________________.

Implementation

19. List some healthy lifestyle measures that contribute to a healthy self-concept.

____

____

____

____

20. In acute care, the nurse is likely to encounter clients who experience ______________________ to their self-concept because of the nature of the treatment and diagnostic procedure.

21. Identify ways a nurse can assist a client in the adjustment to a change in physical appearance.

____

____

____

____

22. Identify teaching strategies to help a client attain a more positive self-concept.

a. ____

b. ____

c. ____

d. ____

e. ____

f. ____

g. ____

h. ____

Evaluation

23. Client care evaluates the actual care delivered by the health team based on expected outcomes. Briefly explain the expected outcomes for a self-concept disturbance.

____

____

____

____

24. Explain how you can facilitate evaluation from a client's perspective.

____

____

REVIEW QUESTIONS

Select the appropriate answer, and cite the rationale for choosing that particular answer.

1. Which of Erikson's developmental stages specifically addresses identity development?
   a. 1–3 years
   b. 3–6 years
   c. 6–12 years
   d. 12–20 years

Answer: ______________ Rationale: ______________

____

____

2. Which of the following statements about body image is correct?
   a. Physical changes are quickly incorporated into a person's body image.
   b. Body image refers only to the external appearance of a person's body.
   c. Body image involves attitudes related to the body, including physical appearance, structure, or function.
   d. Perceptions by other persons have no influence on a person's body image.

Answer: ______________ Rationale: ______________

____

____

3. Sandeep, who is 2 years old, is praised for using his potty instead of wetting his pants. This is an example of learning a behaviour through which of the following?
   a. Identification
   b. Imitation
   c. Substitution
   d. Reinforcement–extinction

Copyright © 2019 Elsevier Canada, a division of Reed Elsevier Canada, Ltd.

Answer:______________ Rationale:______________
____
____

4. Mrs. Watson has just undergone a radical mastectomy. You are aware that Mrs. Watson will probably have considerable anxiety over which of the following?
   a. Role performance
   b. Self-identity
   c. Body image
   d. Self-esteem

Answer:______________ Rationale:______________
____
____

5. Which of the following statements demonstrates that your self-concept is positively affecting the client?
   a. "You've got to take a more active part in caring for your ostomy."
   b. "I know your ostomy is difficult to look at, but you will get used to it in time."
   c. (While grimacing) "Ostomy care isn't so bad."
   d. "Let me show you how to place the bag on your stoma."

Answer:______________ Rationale:______________
____
____

CRITICAL THINKING MODEL FOR NURSING CARE PLAN FOR DISTURBED BODY IMAGE

Imagine that you are the student nurse in the Nursing Care Plan on pages 470–471 of your text. Complete the *assessment phase* of the critical thinking model by writing in the appropriate boxes on the model shown. Think about the following:

- In developing Ms. Johnson's plan of care, what knowledge did you apply?
- In what way might your previous experience apply in this case?
- What intellectual or professional standards were applied to Ms. Johnson?
- What critical thinking attitudes were used in assessing Ms. Johnson?
- As you review your assessment, what key areas did you cover?

Copyright © 2019 Elsevier Canada, a division of Reed Elsevier Canada, Ltd.

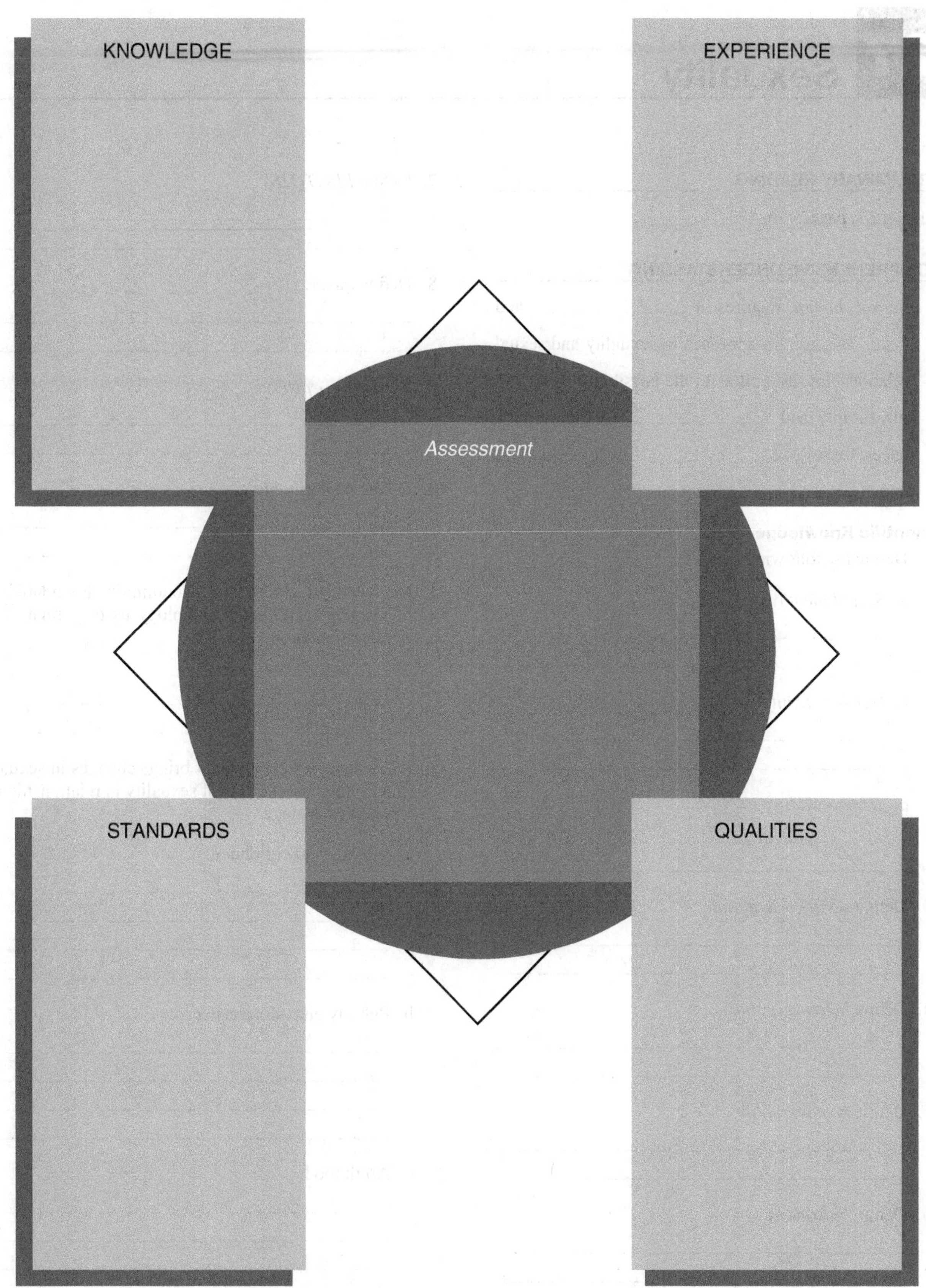

CHAPTER 26 Critical Thinking Model for Nursing Care Plan for *Disturbed Body Image*
See answers on Evolve site.

Copyright © 2019 Elsevier Canada, a division of Reed Elsevier Canada, Ltd.

27 Sexuality

PRELIMINARY READING

Chapter 27, pages 476–493

COMPREHENSIVE UNDERSTANDING

1. *Sexual health* requires a ______________ and ______________ approach to sexuality and sexual relationships, as well as to the possibility of having pleasurable and ______________ sexual experiences, free of______________, ______________, and ______________________________.

Scientific Knowledge Base

2. Define the following:

   a. *Sexual identity*:

   ____

   ____

   b. *Gender identity*:

   ____

   ____

   c. *Transsexuality*:

   ____

   ____

3. Define *sexual orientation.*

____

____

4. Define *heterosexuality.*

____

____

5. Define *homosexuality.*

____

____

6. Define *bisexuality.*

____

____

7. Define *LBGTQ2S.*

____

____

8. Define *queer.*

____

____

9. Define *two-spirited.*

____

____

10. Define *homophobia.*

____

____

11. Describe guidelines from Community Foundations of Canada regarding terminology as they relate to sexual orientation.

____

____

____

12. Each stage of development brings changes in sexual functioning and the role of sexuality in relationships. Explain each stage.

   a. Infancy and childhood:

   ____

   ____

   ____

   ____

   b. Puberty and adolescence:

   ____

   ____

   ____

   ____

   c. Adulthood:

   ____

   ____

   ____

   ____

Copyright © 2019 Elsevier Canada, a division of Reed Elsevier Canada, Ltd.

d. Older personhood:

____

____

____

____

13. The four phases of the *sexual response cycle* are

_______________, _______________, _______________,

and _______________.

14. These phases are the result of vasocongestion and muscle contraction. Explain the physiologic responses for each of the four phases.

a. Female:

____

____

b. Male:

____

____

15. Define *safer sex*.

____

____

16. List three factors that contribute to unsafe sex, especially among adolescents.

a. _______________

b. _______________

c. _______________

17. A major problem in dealing with *sexually transmitted infections (STIs)* is _______________

_______________.

18. List the prevalent STIs.

a. _______________

b. _______________

c. _______________

d. _______________

e. _______________

f. _______________

19. People most likely to contract an STI are those who:

a. _______________

b. _______________

c. _______________

d. _______________

20. Condoms reduce the risk of most STIs (including HIV infection). A condom acts as a barrier to keep

_______________, _______________, and _______________

from passing from one person to another.

21. Numerous contraceptive options are available. Briefly list the options available under the following categories.

a. Nonprescriptive methods:

____

____

b. Methods requiring a health care provider's intervention:

____

____

22. Emergency contraception pills are most effective up

to _______________ hours following intercourse

and are recommended to _______________.

Nursing Knowledge Base

Global cultural diversity creates considerable variability in sexual norms and represents a wide spectrum of beliefs and values.

23. Common areas of sociocultural diversity in sexual behaviour include the following:

a. _______________

b. _______________

c. _______________

d. _______________

e. _______________

24. What might prevent a nurse from discussing issues of sexuality with a patient?

____

25. Explain the following issues.

a. *Infertility*:

____

____

b. *Sexual abuse*:

____

____

c. *Sexual dysfunction*:

____

____

Copyright © 2019 Elsevier Canada, a division of Reed Elsevier Canada, Ltd.

26. Describe the possible sexual concerns that should be considered for each of the following patients.

a. Pregnant and postpartum women:

b. Patients recovering from surgery:

c. Patients with illness or disabilities:

Critical Thinking

27. To care for a patient related to sexuality, a nurse must have a good understanding of ______, ______, ______, and ______, as well as ______.

Sexuality and the Nursing Process

A person's sexuality has physical, psychologic, social, and cultural elements.

Assessment

28. Explain approaches to communication that are useful in eliciting a sexual history from an adult.

Sexual health history

29. List the five *P*s you may use to elicit a brief sexual history from an adult.

a.

b.

c.

d.

e.

30. Briefly explain the physical assessment in evaluating the cause of sexual concerns or problems.

Nursing Diagnosis

31. Identify clues that may signal risk for or an actual nursing diagnosis related to sexuality.

a.

b.

c.

d.

e.

Planning

32. The "PLISSIT" model developed by Annon (1974) guides the planning phases. Explain each of the following parts of the abbreviation.

a. *P*:

b. *LI*:

c. *SS*:

d. *IT*:

Implementation

33. Topics of education vary depending on the defining characteristics and related factors. Describe some situations.

34. Nursing interventions that address alterations in sexuality are aimed at ______, ______, ______, or ______.

35. Identify situational and developmental crises that prompt education.

Copyright © 2019 Elsevier Canada, a division of Reed Elsevier Canada, Ltd.

Evaluation

Patient expectations

36. Patient expectations evaluate care from the patient's perspective. Briefly explain the patient's perspective with respect to resolution of his or her sexual concerns.

REVIEW QUESTIONS

Select the appropriate answer, and cite the rationale for choosing that particular answer.

1. Sexual development in very young children is influenced by which of the following?
   a. Frequent exposure to persons with various sexual orientations
   b. Comfort of parents in communicating about genital parts and personal space
   c. Television and social media that depict gender roles
   d. Sexual behaviours and attitudes of peers

Answer:______________ Rationale:______________

2. Difficulties in finding and treating persons with STIs can be attributed to which of the following? *(Select all that apply.)*
   a. Symptoms go unnoticed
   b. Embarrassment to discuss symptoms
   c. Reluctance to discuss sexual behaviours that may not be seen as "normal"
   d. Popularization by social media of the importance of having multiple sexual partners

Answer:______________ Rationale:______________

3. Why is it often more difficult to discuss sexuality issues with older patients?
   a. Older people are less likely to be sexually active.
   b. They are more likely to have complex causes for sexual problems.
   c. They may have more difficulty discussing intimate issues.
   d. They are frequently deaf, and it is difficult to talk about this in a loud voice.

Answer:______________ Rationale:______________

4. Which processes were not implicated in the sexual response cycle put forth by Masters and Johnson?
   a. Vasoconstriction
   b. Muscle contractions
   c. Desire
   d. Influence of media

Answer:______________ Rationale:______________

5. Your friend maintains that the genitalia you have at birth is not what makes you who you are. Rather, it is how you view yourself that makes you male, female, or some combination. To which of the following is your friend referring?
   a. Gender identity
   b. Bisexuality
   c. Two-spirited
   d. Sexual identity

Answer:______________ Rationale:______________

CRITICAL THINKING MODEL FOR NURSING CARE PLAN FOR SEXUAL DYSFUNCTION

Imagine that you are Jack, the nursing student in the Nursing Care Plan on page 489 of your text. Complete the *assessment* phase of the critical thinking model by writing your answers in the appropriate boxes of the model shown. Think about the following:

- In developing Mr. Clements's plan of care, what knowledge did you apply?
- In what way might your previous experience assist in this case?
- What intellectual or professional standards were applied in caring for Mr. Clements?
- What critical thinking attitudes did you utilize in assessing Mr. Clements?
- As you review your assessment, what key areas did you cover?

Copyright © 2019 Elsevier Canada, a division of Reed Elsevier Canada, Ltd.

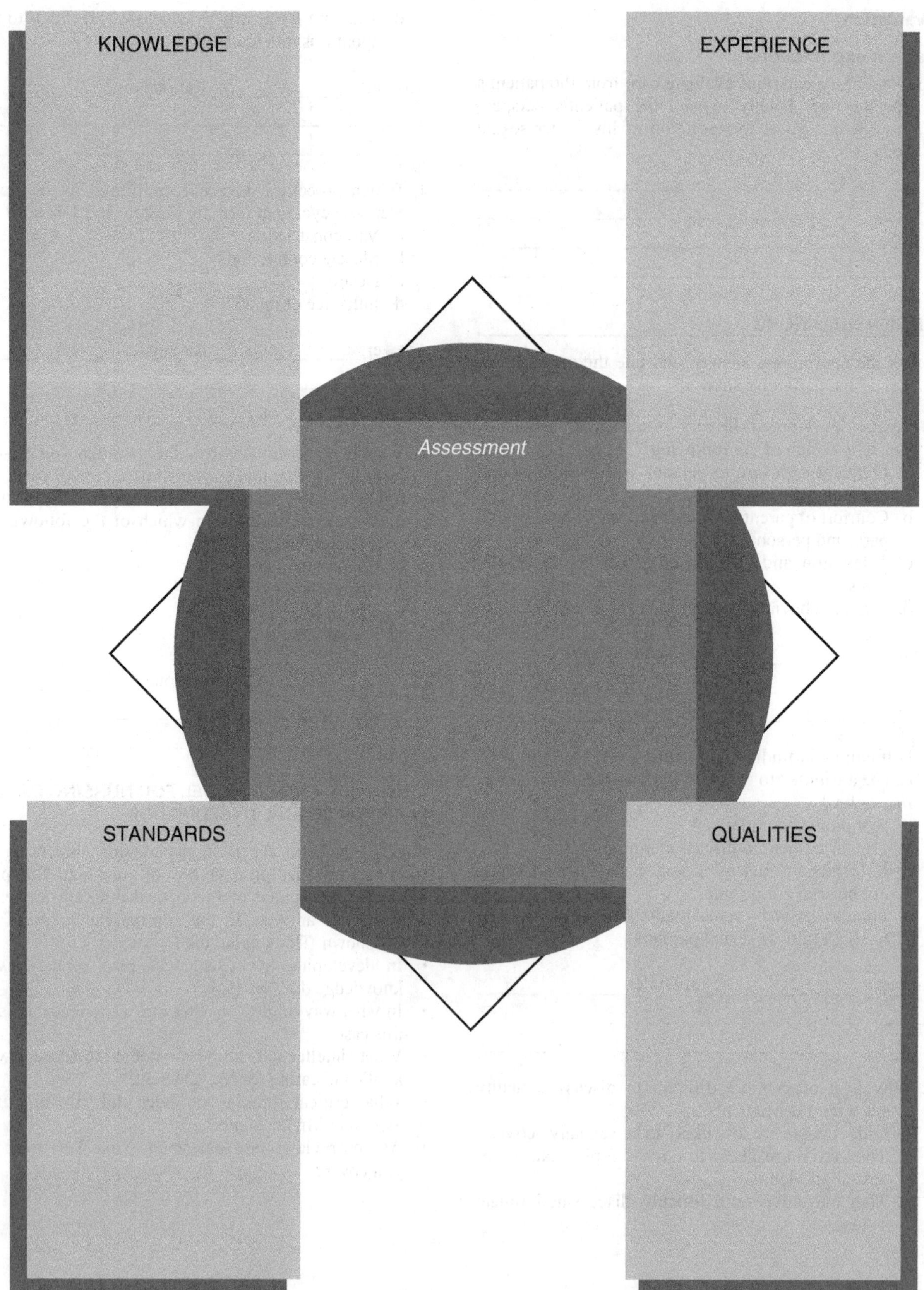

CHAPTER 27 Critical Thinking Model for Nursing Care Plan for *Sexual Dysfunction*
See answers on Evolve site.

Copyright © 2019 Elsevier Canada, a division of Reed Elsevier Canada, Ltd.

28 Spirituality in Health and Health Care

PRELIMINARY READING

Chapter 28, pages 494–507

COMPREHENSIVE UNDERSTANDING

1. Define *spirituality.*

____

____

____

2. Describe the association between spirituality and health.

____

____

____

Historical Perspectives

3. Identify four historical milestones related to spirituality and nursing.

____

____

____

____

Spirituality and Health: Empirical Evidence

4. There is increasing evidence that spirituality plays a role in _______________, _______________, and _______________.

Spirituality and Nursing Theory

5. _______________ was not explicitly addressed in many early nursing models.

6. Thinking about the environment surrounding nursing practice led naturally to _______________ _______________.

7. Dignity is a critical part of _______________ _______________.

Conceptualizing Spirituality and Religion

8. Identify the common themes of spirituality in health care.

____

____

9. Discuss the challenge of defining spirituality for nursing.

____

____

10. Explain the differences between the terms *spirituality* and *religion.*

____

____

____

____

____

11. Explain the concept of *faith.*

____

____

____

12. The belief that comes with faith involves _______________, or an awareness of that which one cannot see or know in ordinary ways.

13. Explain how the following view spirituality.

a. *Atheists*:

____

____

b. *Agnostics*:

____

____

Spirituality and the Life Journey

14. The spirituality of children develops as they _______________ _______________.

15. Evidence of healthy spirituality is _______________ for others and oneself.

16. A _______________ in older persons is one that gives _______________ and _______________.

Copyright © 2019 Elsevier Canada, a division of Reed Elsevier Canada, Ltd.

17. Briefly explain how each of the following may impact a patient's spiritual journey.

    a. Unexpected or chronic illness: ______________________________

    ____

    ____

    b. Terminal illness:

    ____

    ____

    ____

18. Briefly discuss what patients expect from nurses regarding their spiritual care.

    ____

    ____

    ____

    ____

Critical Thinking

19. The nurse's approach to spirituality begins with ______________________.

Understanding patients' spirituality

20. Spiritual care is ______________ from the ______________ aspects of care. Spirituality contains an element of ______________ that cannot be ______________ and ______________ in the same way that you might treat a physical problem. ______________ and ______________ in a patient's spirituality may be considered ______________ and ______________.

21. Describe the nurse's role in understanding a patient's spirituality.

    ____

    ____

    ____

    ____

22. What are the components included in the mnemonic *SACR-D*?

    ____

    ____

23. Discuss the purpose of *spiritual screening.*

    ____

    ____

24. Identify six ways to try to understand a patient's spirituality.

    a. ______________________________

    b. ______________________________

    c. ______________________________

    d. ______________________________

    e. ______________________________

    f. ______________________________

Ethical spiritual care

Discrimination is not a conscious process, but an unchallenged set of biases that cause us to react to others in less than caring ways.

An important part of ethical spiritual care is constantly working with your own potential biases as a nurse.

25. Describe the importance of *reflective practice.*

    ____

    ____

26. Identify two ethical issues that emerge when nurses engage in spiritual care.

    ____

    ____

27. Discuss how the *Code of Ethics for Registered Nurses* can be applied to boundaries and the provision of spiritual care.

    ____

    ____

28. Competencies for spiritual care include ______________

    ____

    ______________________________.

    Although nurses can provide a caring context for patients' spirituality, this should not in any way be misconstrued to suggest that nurses have expertise in spiritual care.

29. Describe how nurses are prepared to provide a good context for spiritual care.

    ____

    ____

    ____

    ____

There is great variability even among common religions, and individuals will pick and choose the practices they adhere to within that religion. You need not be afraid to ask. Many religious individuals will gladly talk about their faith and practices if you are open.

Copyright © 2019 Elsevier Canada, a division of Reed Elsevier Canada, Ltd.

Providing Spiritual Care

30. Spiritual care is often overlooked in the provision of nursing care. Identify some perceived barriers to nurses offering spiritual care.
    a. ____________
    b. ____________
    c. ____________
    d. ____________

31. Spiritual nursing care, at its foundation, is ____________ ____________.

32. Briefly describe *spiritual care.*
    ____
    ____
    ____

33. The ____________ that undergird all of nursing practice are the same skills that create the ____________ ____________.

Facilitating spiritual practices

Rituals that bring meaning to life are spiritual practices. They are integrated throughout a person's daily activities.

34. Give three examples of how a nurse can facilitate spiritual care.
    ____
    ____
    ____

Reflecting on Nurses' Spiritual Care

Scholars have proposed that it is not normally within the nursing role to "evaluate" whether patients achieve connectedness, meaning, peace, hope, or other indicators of spirituality.

35. Identify six spiritual "interventions."
    a. ____________
    b. ____________
    c. ____________
    d. ____________
    e. ____________
    f. ____________

Nurses need to be cautious about entering into the areas of mystery, particularly if we are sensing our own need to explain or control patients' suffering.

REVIEW QUESTIONS

Select the appropriate answer, and cite the rationale for choosing that particular answer.

1. When planning care to include spiritual needs for a patient of the Hindu faith, the religious practices you should understand include all of the following, *except:*
   a. Public prayer is important.
   b. Modesty is important.
   c. Religious symbols should not be removed.
   d. Same-sex caregivers are preferred.

Answer: ____________ Rationale: ____________
____
____

2. The role of the nurse in spiritual care is to do which of the following?
   a. Assess, diagnose, and treat
   b. Delve into the intimate layers of spirituality
   c. Seek to understand and become a co-learner
   d. Not discuss spirituality but refer to religious leaders

Answer: ____________ Rationale: ____________
____
____

3. A patient who practices Judaism may engage in which of the following?
   a. Keep a cross and prayer beads at bedside
   b. Refuse treatment on the Sabbath
   c. Prefer to have pork with meals
   d. Choose death over breaking kosher

Answer: ____________ Rationale: ____________
____
____

4. Which of the following most accurately describes spirituality?
   a. Defined by the individual
   b. The same as religion
   c. An organized system of beliefs
   d. Important to agnostics

Answer: ____________ Rationale: ____________
____
____

Copyright © 2019 Elsevier Canada, a division of Reed Elsevier Canada, Ltd.

5. Mr. Lanois is 90 years old and recently received a diagnosis of a malignant tumour. Staff members have observed him crying on several occasions, and now he cries as he reads from his Bible. Interventions to help Mr. Lanois cope with his illness would include which of the following?
   a. Asking the parish nurse from his congregation to visit him
   b. Engaging Mr. Lanois in diversional activities to reduce feelings of hopelessness
   c. Discouraging family from being involved in activities and planning
   d. Praying with Mr. Lanois as often as possible

Answer: ______________ Rationale: ______________
____
____

Copyright © 2019 Elsevier Canada, a division of Reed Elsevier Canada, Ltd.

29 Stress and Adaptation

PRELIMINARY READING

Chapter 29, pages 508–525

COMPREHENSIVE UNDERSTANDING

1. Define the term *stress*.

______

______

2. *Stressors* are ______

______.

Conceptualizations of Stress

3. Explain the *fight-or-flight* response to stress.

______

______

______

4. List (in sequence) and briefly describe the three stages of the *general adaptation syndrome*.

    a. ______

    ______

    b. ______

    ______

    c. ______

    ______

5. Define *homeostasis*.

______

______

6. Explain the following terms.

    a. *Primary appraisal*:

    ______

    ______

    b. *Secondary appraisal*:

    ______

    ______

    c. *Coping*:

    ______

    ______

7. If previous ways of coping are not effective, a crisis may occur, in which the person faces a turning point in life and the person must change. Give examples of the two types of crisis.

    a. *Developmental crisis*:

    ______

    ______

    b. *Situational crisis*:

    ______

    ______

Stress Response Systems

8. Explain how the following areas of the brain are involved in the stress response.

    a. Reticular formation:

    ______

    ______

    b. Limbic system:

    ______

    ______

    c. Midbrain and pons:

    ______

    ______

    d. Medulla oblongata:

    ______

    ______

9. Describe the activation process of the *HPA axis*.

______

______

______

______

10. Briefly describe the areas of the brain involved in the stress response system.

    a. ______

    ______

    b. ______

    ______

    c. ______

    ______

Copyright © 2019 Elsevier Canada, a division of Reed Elsevier Canada, Ltd.

Stress and the Immune System

11. Dysregulation or chronic activation of the SAM system and the HPA axis may increase the risk of stress-related ______

The Relationship Between Type of Stressor and Health

12. Distinguish between the different types of stress.
   a. *Eustress*:
   b. *Distress*:
   c. *Trauma*:
   d. *Post-traumatic growth*:

13. Stressful events like ______ continue to be prevalent for ______ women.

14. Explain the following stress-related disorders.
   a. *Acute stress disorder*:
   b. *Post-traumatic stress disorder (PTSD)*:

Nursing Knowledge Base

15. Summarize the following models related to stress and coping.
   a. Neuman's systems model:
   b. Pender et al.'s health promotion model:

16. The following factors can potentially be stressors. Explain.
   a. Situational factors:
   b. Maturational factors:
   c. Sociocultural factors:

Critical Thinking

17. Explain the importance of being confident in skills and knowledge when guiding a patient through a stressful situation.

Nursing Process

Assessment

18. Give an example of each of the following subjective factors to assess.
   a. Perception of stressor:
   b. Available coping resources:
   c. Maladaptive coping used:
   d. Adherence to healthy practices:

Copyright © 2019 Elsevier Canada, a division of Reed Elsevier Canada, Ltd.

19. Identify seven objective indicators of stress.
    a. ______
    b. ______
    c. ______
    d. ______
    e. ______
    f. ______
    g. ______

Nursing Diagnosis

20. Give two examples of nursing diagnostic statements related to stress.

______

______

Planning

21. What are the desirable outcomes for persons experiencing stress?
    a. ______
    b. ______
    c. ______
    d. ______

Implementation

22. Identify the primary modes of intervention for stress.
    a. ______
    b. ______
    c. ______

23. Explain how the following methods reduce stressors.
    a. Regular exercise:
    ______
    b. Support systems:
    ______
    c. Time management:
    ______
    d. Guided imagery and visualization:
    ______
    e. Progressive muscle relaxation:
    ______
    f. Assertiveness training:
    ______
    g. Journal writing:
    ______
    h. Stress management in your workplace:
    ______

24. Crises occur when stress overwhelms ______.

25. *Crisis intervention* is ______.

26. Briefly explain when recovery from stress occurs.

______

Evaluation

27. Briefly explain the patient's care in relation to the patient's expectations.

______

REVIEW QUESTIONS

Select the appropriate answer, and cite the rationale for choosing that particular answer.

1. Which definition *does not* characterize stress?
    a. Any situation in which a nonspecific demand requires an individual to respond or take action
    b. A phenomenon affecting social, psychologic, developmental, spiritual, and physiologic dimensions
    c. A condition eliciting an intellectual, behavioural, or metabolic response
    d. Efforts to maintain relative constancy within the internal environment

Answer:______ Rationale:______

Copyright © 2019 Elsevier Canada, a division of Reed Elsevier Canada, Ltd.

2. Which statement about homeostasis is *not* accurate?
   a. Homeostatic mechanisms provide long-term and short-term control over the body's equilibrium.
   b. Homeostatic mechanisms are self-regulatory.
   c. Homeostatic mechanisms function through negative feedback.
   d. Illness may inhibit normal homeostatic mechanisms.

Answer:______________ Rationale:______________

3. Major homeostatic mechanisms are controlled by all of the following *except* which one?
   a. Thymus gland
   b. Medulla oblongata
   c. Reticular formation
   d. Pituitary gland

Answer:______________ Rationale:______________

4. Which of the following is a stage of the general adaptation syndrome?
   a. Alarm reaction
   b. Fight-or-flight response
   c. Coping mechanisms
   d. Inflammatory response

Answer:______________ Rationale:______________

5. Crisis intervention is a specific measure used for helping a patient resolve a particular, immediate stress problem. This approach is based on which of the following?
   a. The ability of the nurse to solve the patient's problems
   b. An in-depth analysis of a patient's situation
   c. Teaching the patient how to help make the mental connection between the stressful event and his or her reaction to it
   d. Effective communication between the nurse and the patient

Answer:______________ Rationale:______________

CRITICAL THINKING MODEL FOR NURSING CARE PLAN FOR CAREGIVER ROLE STRAIN

Imagine that you are the student nurse in the Nursing Care Plan on pages 518–519 of your text. Complete the *evaluation* phase of the critical thinking model by writing your answers in the appropriate boxes of the model shown. Think about the following:

- In evaluating the care of Carl and Evelyn, what knowledge did you apply?
- In what way might your previous experience influence the evaluation of Carl's care?
- During evaluation, what intellectual and professional standards were applied to Carl's care?
- In what way do critical thinking attitudes play a role in how you approach the evaluation of Carl's care?

Copyright © 2019 Elsevier Canada, a division of Reed Elsevier Canada, Ltd.

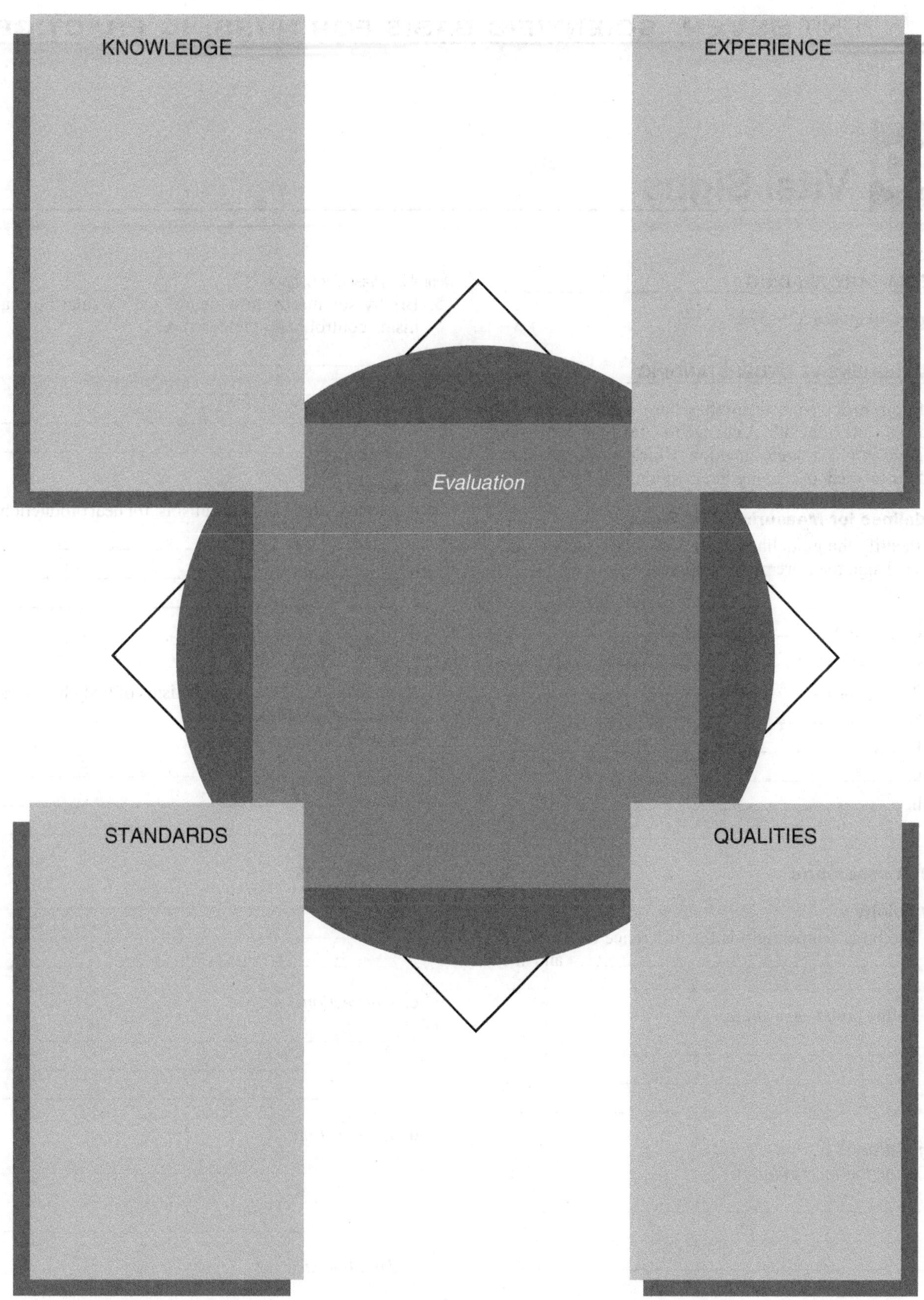

CHAPTER 29 Critical Thinking Model for Nursing Care Plan for *Caregiver Role Strain*
See answers on Evolve site.

Copyright © 2019 Elsevier Canada, a division of Reed Elsevier Canada, Ltd.

UNIT **SEVEN** SCIENTIFIC BASIS FOR NURSING PRACTICE

30 Vital Signs

PRELIMINARY READING

Chapter 30, pages 526–574

COMPREHENSIVE UNDERSTANDING

Vital signs provide important (baseline) data to determine the usual state of health. A change in vital signs indicates a change in physiologic function, which may signal the need for medical or nursing intervention.

Guidelines for Measuring Vital Signs

1. Identify the guidelines that assist you to incorporate vital sign measurement into practice.
   a. ______
   b. ______
   c. ______
   d. ______
   e. ______
   f. ______
   g. ______
   h. ______
   i. ______

Body Temperature

Physiology

2. The body temperature is the difference between the ______ and the ______.

3. Define *core temperature.*

______

Regulation

4. Define *thermoregulation.*

______

Neural and Vascular Control.

5. Briefly summarize how neural and vascular mechanisms control body temperature.

______

Heat Production.

6. List four sources, or mechanisms, for heat production.
   a. ______
   b. ______
   c. ______
   d. ______

Heat Loss.

7. Explain the following mechanisms of body heat loss, and give an example of each.
   a. *Radiation*:
   ______
   b. *Conduction*:
   ______
   c. *Convection*:
   ______
   d. *Evaporation*:
   ______
   e. *Diaphoresis*:
   ______

Copyright © 2019 Elsevier Canada, a division of Reed Elsevier Canada, Ltd.

Skin in Temperature Regulation.

8. Briefly explain the skin's role in temperature regulation.
   a. Insulation of the body:
   b. Vasoconstriction:
   c. Temperature sensation:

Behavioural Control.

9. Identify four factors that must be present for a person to control body temperature.
   a.
   b.
   c.
   d.

Factors affecting body temperature

10. Changes in body temperature within the normal range occur when the relationship between heat production and heat loss is altered by physiologic or behavioural variables. Summarize the following variables.
    a. Age:
    b. Exercise:
    c. Hormone level:
    d. Circadian rhythm:
    e. Stress:
    f. Environment:

Temperature Alterations

11. Temperature alterations can be related to _____, _____, _____, _____, or any combination of these alterations.

Fever.

12. *Pyrexia*, or *fever*, occurs because _____.
13. Explain how a fever works as an important defence mechanism.
14. Explain how a fever serves a diagnostic purpose.
15. Explain how a fever affects metabolism.

Hyperthermia.

16. Define the following terms.
    a. *Hyperthermia*:
    b. *Malignant hyperthermia*:

Heatstroke.

17. Define *heatstroke* and identify its signs and symptoms.

Copyright © 2019 Elsevier Canada, a division of Reed Elsevier Canada, Ltd.

Heat Exhaustion.

18. Define *heat exhaustion* and identify treatments.

Hypothermia.

19. Define *hypothermia* and identify causes.

20. *Frostbite* occurs when ______.

Assessment

Sites

21. List the routine assessment sites for intermittent temperature measurement (both invasively and noninvasively).
    a.
    b.
    c.
    d.
    e.
    f.

Thermometers

22. Identify three types of thermometers, and list advantages and disadvantages of each.
    a.
    b.
    c.

Nursing Diagnosis

23. Identify four nursing diagnoses related to *thermoregulation*.
    a.
    b.
    c.
    d.

Planning

Match patients' needs with interventions that are supported and recommended in the clinical research literature.

Implementation

Health promotion

24. Health promotion for patients at risk of altered temperature is directed toward ______.

25. Identify those who are at risk for hypothermia.

Acute care

Fever

The procedures used to intervene and treat an elevated temperature depend on the fever's cause; its adverse effects; and its strength, intensity, and duration of the elevation.

26. Explain the differences related to febrile states in each of the following:
    a. Children:
    b. Hypersensitivity to medications:

27. Give four examples of each type of fever therapy.

    Pharmacologic:
    a.
    b.
    c.
    d.

    Nonpharmacologic:
    a.
    b.
    c.
    d.

28. Describe a nursing intervention to control shivering.

Copyright © 2019 Elsevier Canada, a division of Reed Elsevier Canada, Ltd.

Heatstroke

29. Initial treatment for heatstroke includes ________, ________, ________, and ________.

Hypothermia

30. Summarize the treatment for hypothermia (both in and away from the health care setting).

Restorative and continuing care

31. Summarize the patient teaching in regard to the treatment of a fever.

Evaluation

Pulse

32. Define *pulse.*

Physiology and regulation

33. Define the following terms.
   a. *Stroke volume*:
   b. *Cardiac output*:

Assessment of pulse

34. Identify the two most common pulse sites assessed by nurses.
   a. ________
   b. ________

Use of a Stethoscope

35. Identify the five major parts of the stethoscope.
   a. ________
   b. ________
   c. ________
   d. ________
   e. ________

Character of the pulse

36. List four characteristics to identify during peripheral pulse assessment. Using an asterisk, specify the two characteristics to identify when assessing an apical pulse.
   a. ________
   b. ________
   c. ________
   d. ________

37. Define the following terms.
   a. *Tachycardia*:
   b. *Bradycardia*:
   c. *Pulse deficit*:
   d. *Dysrhythmia*:

Respiration

38. Define the following terms.
   a. *Ventilation*:
   b. *Diffusion*:

Copyright © 2019 Elsevier Canada, a division of Reed Elsevier Canada, Ltd.

c. *Perfusion*:

Physiologic control

Breathing is a passive process. The respiratory centre in the brainstem regulates the involuntary control of respirations.

39. Ventilation is regulated by levels of ______________, ______________, and ______________ in the arterial blood.

40. The most important factor in the control of ventilation is the level of ______________.

41. *Hypoxemia* occurs when ______________.

Mechanics of breathing

42. Briefly summarize the process of *inspiration*.

43. Define the following terms.

a. *Tidal volume*:

b. *Eupnea*:

Assessment of ventilation

44. Accurate measurement of ventilation requires ______________ and ______________ movements.

45. List three objective measurements used in respiratory status assessment.

a.
b.
c.

46. Define the following alterations in breathing patterns.

a. Bradypnea:

b. Tachypnea:

c. Hyperpnea:

d. Apnea:

e. Hyperventilation:

f. Hypoventilation:

g. Cheyne-Stokes respiration:

h. Kussmaul respiration:

i. Biot respiration:

Assessment of diffusion and perfusion

The respiratory processes of diffusion and perfusion can be evaluated by measuring the oxygen saturation of the blood.

47. The percentage of oxygen saturation of arterial blood is ______________ and of venous blood is ______________.

Measurement of Arterial Oxygen Saturation

48. Explain the purpose of a *pulse oximeter*.

49. List two factors that can affect the accuracy of an oxygen saturation reading.

a.
b.

Copyright © 2019 Elsevier Canada, a division of Reed Elsevier Canada, Ltd.

Blood Pressure

50. Define the following terms.
    a. *Blood pressure*: ____________________
    ____
    b. *Systolic*: ____________________
    ____
    c. *Diastolic*: ____________________
    ____

51. The difference between the systolic and diastolic pressure is the ____________________.

Physiology of arterial blood pressure

52. Blood pressure reflects the interrelationships of the following. Briefly explain each.
    a. Cardiac output: ____________________
    ____
    ____
    b. Peripheral vascular resistance: ____________________
    ____
    ____
    c. Blood volume: ____________________
    ____
    ____
    d. Blood viscosity: ____________________
    ____
    ____
    e. Artery elasticity: ____________________
    ____
    ____

Factors influencing blood pressure

53. List six factors that influence blood pressure.
    a. ____________________
    b. ____________________
    c. ____________________
    d. ____________________
    e. ____________________
    f. ____________________

Hypertension

54. Identify the criteria for the diagnosis of hypertension in an adult.
    ____
    ____
    ____
    ____

55. Briefly summarize the physiology of hypertension.
    ____
    ____
    ____
    ____

56. List six risk factors that are linked to hypertension.
    a. ____________________
    b. ____________________
    c. ____________________
    d. ____________________
    e. ____________________
    f. ____________________

Hypotension

57. Identify the criteria for the diagnosis of hypotension in an adult.
    ____
    ____
    ____
    ____

58. Explain the physiology of hypotension and its causes.
    ____
    ____
    ____
    ____

59. Orthostatic hypotension, also known as ____________________, occurs when ____________________.

Copyright © 2019 Elsevier Canada, a division of Reed Elsevier Canada, Ltd.

60. Explain how you would assess a patient for orthostatic hypotension.

______

______

______

______

Measurement of blood pressure

61. Identify two methods for measuring blood pressure.

a. ______

______

b. ______

______

Blood Pressure Equipment

62. Identify the two types of manometers used in *sphygmomanometers*, and list their advantages and disadvantages.

a. ______

______

______

______

b. ______

______

______

______

Auscultation

63. Identify common mistakes in blood pressure assessment.

a. ______

b. ______

c. ______

d. ______

e. ______

f. ______

g. ______

h. ______

i. ______

j. ______

k. ______

l. ______

m. ______

n. ______

64. During the initial assessment, you should obtain and record the blood pressure in both arms. Pressure differences between the arms greater than ______ mm Hg indicate vascular problems.

65. The sounds heard over an artery distal to the blood pressure cuff are Korotkoff sounds. Describe each.

a. First:

______

______

b. Second:

______

______

c. Third:

______

______

d. Fourth:

______

______

e. Fifth:

______

______

Assessment in Children

66. Identify four reasons why the measurement of blood pressure in infants and children is difficult.

a. ______

b. ______

c. ______

d. ______

Ultrasonic Stethoscope

67. Explain the rationale for the use of an ultrasonic stethoscope.

______

______

______

______

Palpation

68. Identify the method you may use to assess blood pressure when Korotkoff sounds are not audible with the standard stethoscope.

______

______

______

______

Copyright © 2019 Elsevier Canada, a division of Reed Elsevier Canada, Ltd.

69. Define *auscultatory gap.*

Lower Extremity Blood Pressure

70. Give an example of when you would assess a patient's blood pressure using the patient's lower extremities.

Automatic Blood Pressure Devices

71. Identify the advantages and disadvantages of using automatic blood pressure devices.

Self-Measurement of Blood Pressure

72. List the benefits of blood pressure self-measurement.
    a.
    b.
    c.
    d.

Recording Vital Signs

73. Identify at least two variations that are unique to the older person.
    a. Temperature:
    b. Pulse rate:
    c. Blood pressure:
    d. Respirations:

REVIEW QUESTIONS

Select the appropriate answer, and cite the rationale for choosing that particular answer.

1. What role does the skin play in temperature regulation?
   a. Insulates the body
   b. Constricts blood vessels
   c. Senses external temperature variations
   d. All of the above

Answer: Rationale:

2. How does minimizing coverings on the body of a patient with a fever promote heat loss?
   a. Radiation, convection, and evaporation
   b. Evaporation
   c. Condensation
   d. Radiation

Answer: Rationale:

3. You are assessing a patient suspected of having the nursing diagnosis *hyperthermia related to vigorous exercise in hot weather.* What is the most important sign of heatstroke?
   a. Confusion
   b. Hot, dry skin
   c. Excess thirst
   d. Muscle cramps

Answer: Rationale:

4. When taking a patient's radial pulse, you note a dysrhythmia. What is the most appropriate action?
   a. Inform the physician immediately
   b. Wait 5 minutes and retake the radial pulse
   c. Take the pulse apically for 1 full minute
   d. Check the patient's record for the presence of a previous dysrhythmia

Answer: Rationale:

5. You are auscultating Mrs. McKinnon's blood pressure. You inflate the cuff to 180 mm Hg. At 156 mm Hg, you hear the onset of a tapping sound. At 130 mm Hg, the sound changes to a murmur or swishing. At 100 mm Hg, the sound momentarily becomes sharper, and at 92 mm Hg, it becomes muffled. At 88 mm Hg, the sound disappears. What is Mrs. McKinnon's blood pressure?
   a. 180/92
   b. 180/130
   c. 156/88
   d. 130/88

Answer: Rationale:

Copyright © 2019 Elsevier Canada, a division of Reed Elsevier Canada, Ltd.

31 Pain Assessment and Management

PRELIMINARY READING

Chapter 31, pages 575–610

COMPREHENSIVE UNDERSTANDING

1. Define *pain.*

Pain is a highly personal experience that can only be accurately described by the individual experiencing it.

Pain and pain management options are viewed within the context of comfort; providing comfort is central to nursing.

The relief from pain is considered a basic human right.

Scientific Knowledge Base

Nature of pain

The nature of the stimulus for pain can be physical, psychologic, or a combination of both.

Physiology of pain

2. Explain the four processes of nociceptive pain.
   a. *Transduction*:
   b. *Transmission*:
   c. *Perception*:
   d. *Modulation*:
3. Explain the two types of neuroregulators.
   a. Neurotransmitters:
   b. Neuromodulators:
4. Identify the neurophysiologic function of the following neuroregulators.
   a. Substance P:
   b. Prostaglandins:
   c. Serotonin:
   d. Endorphins:
   e. Bradykinin:

Theory of Pain

5. Explain the *theory of pain.*

Physiologic Responses

6. List some physiologic responses to pain.
   a. Sympathetic stimulation:
      (i)
      (ii)
      (iii)
      (iv)
      (v)
      (vi)
      (vii)
      (viii)

Copyright © 2019 Elsevier Canada, a division of Reed Elsevier Canada, Ltd.

b. Parasympathetic stimulation:
(i) ________
(ii) ________
(iii) ________
(iv) ________
(v) ________

Behavioural Responses

7. Identify four behavioural changes that characterize a patient experiencing pain.
a. ________
b. ________
c. ________
d. ________

Types of pain

Acute Pain

8. List four characteristics of *acute pain.*
a. ________
b. ________
c. ________
d. ________

Chronic Pain

9. Define *chronic pain.*

____

10. Chronic pain may be ________ or ________.

11. Discuss the impact of chronic noncancer pain.

____

Cancer Pain

Many individuals with cancer pain live in community settings, and pain relief is often provided by their families. Accessing community resources may be difficult for these families, and the stress of caring for a loved one with cancer pain can affect the health of family caregivers.

Pain by Inferred Pathology Process

12. Nociceptive pain is subdivided into ________ and ________ pain. Neuropathic pain arises from ______ or ______ pain nerves.

Breakthrough Pain

13. Define *breakthrough pain.*

____

Nursing Knowledge Base

Knowledge, attitudes, and beliefs

14. Identify common biases and misconceptions about pain.

____

Factors influencing pain

Physiological Factors

Age

15. Explain the developmental differences of the following patients' reaction to pain.
a. Young children:
____
b. Toddlers and preschoolers:
____
c. Older persons:
____

16. Identify any five misconceptions about pain in older patients.
a. ________
b. ________
c. ________
d. ________
e. ________

Sleep

17. Sleep disturbances heighten the perception of pain. Explain.

____

Copyright © 2019 Elsevier Canada, a division of Reed Elsevier Canada, Ltd.

Neurologic Function

18. Explain how a patient's neurologic function can influence pain.

Social Factors

19. Discuss how each of the following influences pain.

a. Attention:

b. Previous experience:

c. Family and social support:

Psychologic Factors

20. Explain how the following psychologic factors affect pain.

a. Anxiety:

b. Meaning of pain:

c. Spiritual factors:

Cultural Factors

21. Explain how cultural factors affect pain.

Nursing Process and Pain

22. Pain management extends beyond pain relief; it encompasses the patient's ____________ and ability to ____________, and to ____________.

Assessment

Pain assessment is the basis of all pain management.

23. Monitor the patient's pain consistently along with other assessments, such as ____________, especially if the pain is not well controlled.

24. Assessment of chronic pain should focus on ____________, ____________, and ____________ dimensions of the pain and on its history and context.

25. Explain what is meant by SMART pain management goals, ____________, and the components used in "OPQRSTUV."

O:

P:

Q:

R:

S:

T:

U:

V:

Expression of pain

Cognitively impaired patients might require simple assessment approaches involving close observation of behaviour changes, especially movement.

Characteristics of pain

26. Briefly explain the common characteristics of pain.

a. Onset, duration, and sequence of pain:

b. Provocation/pain pattern:

Copyright © 2019 Elsevier Canada, a division of Reed Elsevier Canada, Ltd.

c. Palliation/relief measures:

____

____

____

d. Quality:

____

____

____

e. Radiation/location:

____

____

____

f. Severity/intensity:

____

____

____

27. Describe the following scales for measuring the severity of pain.

a. Numerical rating scale:

____

____

b. Verbal descriptor scale:

____

____

c. Visual analogue scale:

____

____

d. FACES scale:

____

____

Contributing Symptoms

28. Identify some contributing symptoms that may aggravate pain.

____

____

____

____

Effects of Pain

29. Pain is a __________, __________, and __________ stressor that ______________________________.

Behavioural Effects/Nonverbal Indicators

30. Give examples of the following behavioural/nonverbal indicators of pain.

a. Vocalizations:

____

____

b. Facial expressions:

____

____

c. Body movement:

____

____

d. Social interaction:

____

____

Influence on Activities of Daily Living

31. Explain how pain can influence activities of daily living in regard to the following:

a. Sleep:

____

____

b. Hygiene:

____

____

c. Sexual relations:

____

____

d. Employment:

____

____

e. Social activities:

____

____

Copyright © 2019 Elsevier Canada, a division of Reed Elsevier Canada, Ltd.

Nursing Diagnosis

The nursing diagnosis focuses on the nature of the pain so that the nurse can identify the best interventions for relieving pain and minimizing its effect on the patient's lifestyle and function.

32. List five potential or actual nursing diagnoses related to a patient in pain.
    a. ______
    b. ______
    c. ______
    d. ______
    e. ______

Planning

Patients in pain frequently have interrelated problems. As one problem worsens, others also change.

Goals and outcomes

33. List the patient outcomes appropriate for the patient experiencing pain.
    a. ______
    b. ______
    c. ______

Setting priorities

Your priorities will change as the patient's pain experience changes.

Implementation

Health promotion

Provide patients and their families with education and information about pain; it will help to reduce anxiety and it increases a patient's sense of control.

34. Describe how you would teach a child about a painful procedure.

______

Nonpharmacologic Pain-Relief Interventions

35. Discuss the goals of the following pain-relief interventions.

    a. Cognitive-behavioural interventions:

    ______

    b. Physical interventions:

    ______

Relaxation and Guided Imagery

36. Briefly explain how *relaxation* lessens pain.

______

37. Briefly explain how the nurse would guide a patient through *progressive relaxation exercises*.

______

38. Briefly explain how the nurse would lead a patient through *guided imagery*.

______

Distraction

39. Define *distraction*, and list one disadvantage and one advantage of using distraction to alleviate perception of pain.

______

40. Describe the effects of using music as a distraction to decrease pain.

______

41. Define the following pain-relief measures and the rationale for their use.

    a. *Biofeedback*:

    ______

    b. *Acupuncture*:

    ______

    c. *Cutaneous stimulation*:

    ______

Copyright © 2019 Elsevier Canada, a division of Reed Elsevier Canada, Ltd.

d. *Herbal supplements*:

____

____

e. *Reducing pain perception*:

____

____

42. What is *TENS*, and how is it believed to reduce pain?

____

____

____

Acute care

Acute Pain Management

The key to pain relief's success is the ongoing evaluation of interventions.

Pharmacologic Pain-Relief Interventions

The ideal analgesic has yet to be developed, but many opioid and nonopioid pain-relieving medications are available.

Analgesics

Analgesics are the most common method of pain relief.

43. Identify the three types of analgesics.

a. _______________

b. _______________

c. _______________

44. Discuss the importance of around-the-clock dosing.

____

____

____

____

Patient-Controlled Analgesia

45. Explain the benefits of patient-controlled analgesia.

____

____

____

____

Local and Regional Anaesthetics and Analgesics

46. Describe what a *local anaesthetic* is, how it may be applied, and possible side effects.

____

____

47. Describe what a *regional anaesthetic* is and list three types.

____

____

____

____

48. Explain an advantage of *epidural analgesia* and how it is administered.

____

____

____

____

Nursing Implications

49. Describe six goals of nursing care for a patient with epidural infusions. Explain one intervention for each goal.

a. _______________

b. _______________

c. _______________

d. _______________

e. _______________

f. _______________

Invasive Interventions for Pain Relief

50. When pain is severe, invasive interventions may give relief when more conservative treatment is neither tolerated nor effective. List any three examples of invasive interventions used to relieve pain.

a. _______________

b. _______________

c. _______________

Procedure pain management

Premedicating patients before painful procedures may assist them to cooperate and may help to reduce the experience of pain.

Cancer Pain Management

51. Identify the three-step approach to cancer pain management recommended by the World Health Organization (1996).

a. _______________

b. _______________

c. _______________

52. Identify patients who are candidates for continuous infusions.

a. _______________

b. _______________

c. _______________

53. Discuss the guidelines for safe administration of morphine sulphate via ambulatory infusion pumps.

____

____

____

Copyright © 2019 Elsevier Canada, a division of Reed Elsevier Canada, Ltd.

Barriers to Effective Pain Management

54. Multiple barriers prevent effective pain management. Identify four barriers for the following categories.

    a. Barriers for patients:

    ______
    ______
    ______
    ______

    b. Barriers for health care providers:

    ______
    ______
    ______
    ______

    c. Barriers for the health care system:

    ______
    ______
    ______
    ______

Restorative and continuing care
Pain Clinics, Palliative Care, and Hospices

55. Briefly discuss the following terms.
    a. *Palliative care*:

    ______

    b. *Hospice care*:

    ______

Evaluation

Patient care

If a patient continues to have discomfort after an intervention, a different approach may be needed. For example, if an analgesic provides only partial relief, the nurse may add relaxation exercises or guided-imagery exercises.

Pain assessment and responses to intervention should be accurately and thoroughly documented so that they can be communicated to others caring for the patient.

Patient perceptions

The patient, if able, is the best judge of whether pain-relief measures work.

The family often is another valuable resource, particularly in the case of the patient with cancer who may not be able to express discomfort during the latter stages of terminal illness.

REVIEW QUESTIONS

Select the appropriate answer, and cite the rationale for choosing that particular answer.

1. What best describes pain as a protective mechanism warning of tissue injury?
   a. Symptom of a severe illness or disease
   b. Subjective experience
   c. Objective experience
   d. Acute symptom of short duration

Answer: ______ Rationale: ______

______

______

2. What is the substance that may cause analgesia when it attaches to opiate receptors in the brain?
   a. Substance P
   b. Serotonin
   c. Prostaglandin
   d. Endorphin

Answer: ______ Rationale: ______

______

______

3. Which question would be appropriate to ask when assessing the quality of a patient's pain?
   a. "Tell me what your pain feels like."
   b. "Is your pain a crushing sensation?"
   c. "How long have you had this pain?"
   d. "Is it a sharp pain or a dull pain?"

Answer: ______ Rationale: ______

______

______

4. Which of the following best describes principles for the use of patient distraction in pain control?
   a. Small C fibres transmit impulses via the spinothalamic tract.
   b. The reticular formation can send inhibitory signals to gating mechanisms.
   c. Large A fibres compete with pain impulses to close gates to painful stimuli.
   d. Transmission of pain impulses from the spinal cord to the cerebral cortex can be inhibited.

Answer: ______ Rationale: ______

______

______

Copyright © 2019 Elsevier Canada, a division of Reed Elsevier Canada, Ltd.

5. What is the best method to use when teaching a child about painful procedures?
   a. Early warnings of the anticipated pain
   b. Storytelling about the upcoming procedure
   c. Relevant play and language directed toward procedure activities
   d. Avoiding explanations until the pain is experienced

Answer: ______________ Rationale: ______________

____

____

CRITICAL THINKING MODEL FOR NURSING CARE PLAN FOR ACUTE PAIN

Imagine that you are the student nurse in the Care Plan on pages 591–593 of your text. Complete the *assessment* phase of the critical thinking model by writing your answers in the appropriate boxes of the model shown. Think about the following:

- What knowledge base is applied to Mrs. Mays?
- In what way might previous experience assist you in this case?
- What intellectual and professional standards were applied to the care of Mrs. Mays?
- What critical thinking attitudes did you use in assessing Mrs. Mays?
- As you review your assessment, what key areas did you cover?

Copyright © 2019 Elsevier Canada, a division of Reed Elsevier Canada, Ltd.

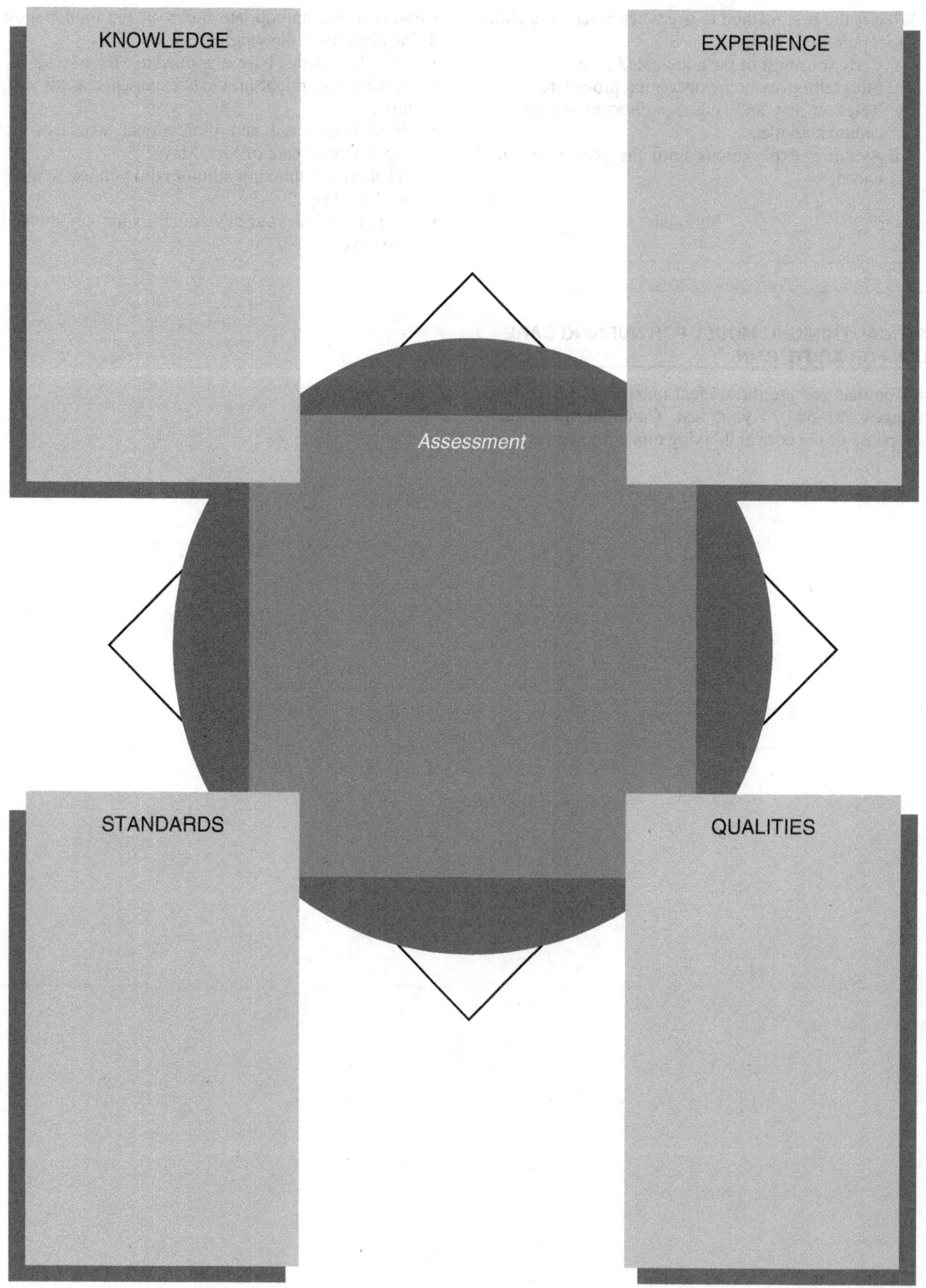

CHAPTER 31 Critical Thinking Model for Nursing Care Plan for *Acute Pain*
See answers on Evolve site.

Copyright © 2019 Elsevier Canada, a division of Reed Elsevier Canada, Ltd.

32 Health Assessment and Physical Examination

PRELIMINARY READING

Chapter 32, pages 611–682

COMPREHENSIVE UNDERSTANDING

Social and Cultural Considerations

Cultural assessment data inform culturally safe physical assessments by providing information that helps the nurse think critically about the political, social, and economic contexts of patients' lives, and how inequities in power and access to resources for health influence the health of individuals.

Purposes of Physical Examination

1. Physical assessment enables the nurse to ________

   and ________________________.

2. List the five nursing purposes for performing a physical assessment.

   a. ________________________

   b. ________________________

   c. ________________________

   d. ________________________

   e. ________________________

Gathering a health history

The main objective of interacting with patients is to find out what their concerns are and to help them find solutions.

Developing nursing diagnoses and a care plan

After gathering information about the patient's health from the health history, a subsequent physical assessment can reveal information that refutes, confirms, or supplements the history.

Skills of Physical Assessment

Inspection

3. Define *inspection.*

   ____

4. List six principles to facilitate accurate inspection of body parts.

   a. ________________________

   b. ________________________

   c. ________________________

   d. ________________________

   e. ________________________

   f. ________________________

Palpation

5. Define *palpation.*

   ____

6. Identify the parts of the hand to use to assess each of the following:

   a. Temperature: ________________

   b. Moisture: ________________

   c. Turgor: ________________

   d. Tenderness and thickness: ________________

Percussion

7. Identify the information obtained through *percussion.*

   ____

Auscultation

8. Define *auscultation.*

   ____

Copyright © 2019 Elsevier Canada, a division of Reed Elsevier Canada, Ltd.

9. Briefly explain the following characteristics of sound.
   a. Frequency: ____________
   b. Loudness: ____________
   c. Quality: ____________
   d. Duration: ____________

Olfaction

While assessing a patient, become familiar with the nature and source of body odours. Olfaction helps to detect abnormalities that you cannot recognize by any other means.

Preparation for the Physical Examination

Infection control

Examination techniques cause the nurse to be in contact with body fluids and discharge. Standard precautions should be used throughout the examination.

Environment

10. List at least three environmental factors that the nurse should attempt to control before performing a physical examination.
    a. ____________
    b. ____________
    c. ____________

Equipment

Hand hygiene is done before equipment preparation and before the examination.

All equipment should be checked to see that it functions properly.

11. Briefly explain the following preexamination preparations.
    a. Physical: ____________
    b. Positioning: ____________
    c. Psychologic: ____________

Assessment of age groups

12. List seven ways to facilitate data collection when examining children.
    a. ____________
    b. ____________
    c. ____________
    d. ____________
    e. ____________
    f. ____________
    g. ____________

Organization of the Examination

13. List eight principles to follow for a well-organized examination.
    a. ____________
    b. ____________
    c. ____________
    d. ____________
    e. ____________
    f. ____________
    g. ____________
    h. ____________

General Survey

General appearance and behaviour

14. List at least eight specific observations of the patient's general appearance and behaviour that should be reviewed.
    a. ____________
    b. ____________
    c. ____________
    d. ____________
    e. ____________
    f. ____________
    g. ____________
    h. ____________

15. Identify the questions related to the following acronym.
    C: ____________
    A: ____________
    G: ____________
    E: ____________

Height and weight

16. List three actions that should be taken to ensure accurate weight measurement of a hospitalized patient.
    a. ____________
    b. ____________
    c. ____________

The Integumentary System—Skin, Hair, and Nails

Skin

17. List the risks for skin lesions that may result in the hospitalized patient.

    ____

Copyright © 2019 Elsevier Canada, a division of Reed Elsevier Canada, Ltd.

18. Define the following terms.

    a. *Melanoma*:

    b. *Pigmentation*:

19. For each skin colour variation, identify in the following table the mechanism that produces colour change, common causes of the variation, and the optimal sites for assessment.

Skin Colour	Condition	Causes	Assessment Locations
Cyanosis (bluish)			
Pallor			
Loss of pigmentation			
Jaundice (yellow-orange)			
Erythema (red)			
Tan-brown			

20. Identify two conditions that are due to excessive skin dryness.

    a.

    b.

The temperature of the skin depends on the amount of blood circulating through the dermis. Increased or decreased skin temperature indicates an increase or decrease in blood flow. Always assess skin temperature for patients at risk of having impaired circulation.

21. Define the following terms.

    a. *Indurated*:

    b. *Turgor*:

    c. *Petechiae:*

    d. *Edema*:

    e. *Senile keratosis*:

    f. *Cherry angiomas*:

22. Briefly describe the following primary skin lesions, and give an example of each.

    a. Macule:

    b. Papule:

    c. Nodule:

    d. Tumour:

    e. Wheal:

    f. Vesicle:

Copyright © 2019 Elsevier Canada, a division of Reed Elsevier Canada, Ltd.

g. Pustule:

h. Ulcer:

i. Atrophy:

Cancerous lesions frequently undergo changes in colour and size. *Report abnormal lesions to the health care provider for further examination.*

Hair and scalp

Inspection

23. Name the three types of lice.

a.

b.

c.

Nails

24. Briefly describe the following abnormalities of the nail bed.

a. Clubbing:

b. Beau lines:

c. Koilonychia:

d. Splinter hemorrhages:

e. Paronychia:

Capillary refill is a test that applies gentle, firm, quick pressure with the thumb to the nail bed; release and observe the results. As you apply pressure, the nail bed will appear white or blanched; however, the pink colour should return immediately on release of pressure. Failure of the pinkness to return promptly indicates circulatory insufficiency.

Head and Neck

Head

25. Define the following head abnormalities.

a. *Hydrocephalus*:

b. *Acromegaly*:

Eyes

26. Define the following common eye and visual abnormalities.

a. Hyperopia:

b. Myopia:

c. Presbyopia:

d. Retinopathy:

e. Strabismus:

f. Amblyopia:

g. Cataracts:

h. Glaucoma:

i. Macular degeneration:

Copyright © 2019 Elsevier Canada, a division of Reed Elsevier Canada, Ltd.

External Eye Structures

27. Examination of the eye includes assessment of five areas. Name them.

a. __________

b. __________

c. __________

d. __________

e. __________

28. Identify the structures of the external eye that you would inspect.

a. __________

b. __________

c. __________

d. __________

e. __________

f. __________

g. __________

29. Define the following terms related to the external eye.

a. *Exophthalmos*:

b. *Ptosis*:

c. *Ectropion*:

d. *Entropion*:

e. *Conjunctivitis*:

f. *Arcus senilis*:

g. *PERRLA*:

Internal Eye Structures

30. Identify the internal eye structures that you would examine with an ophthalmoscope.

Extraocular Movements

As the patient gazes in each direction, observe for parallel eye movement, the position of the upper eyelid in relation to the iris, and the presence of abnormal movements. Disturbances in eye movement reflect local injury to eye muscles and supporting structures or a disorder of the cranial nerves innervating the muscles.

Visual Acuity

31. The assessment of visual acuity, the ability to see small details, tests central vision. Near vision is assessed by __________. Distance vision is assessed using a __________.

Ears

32. Identify the ear structures.

a. __________

b. __________

c. __________

33. List the steps of hearing (sound travelling through the ear by air and bone conduction).

a. __________

b. __________

c. __________

d. __________

e. __________

Hearing Acuity

34. Identify three types of hearing loss.

a. __________

b. __________

c. __________

Nose and sinuses

35. Define the following terms that relate to the nose.

a. *Excoriation*:

Copyright © 2019 Elsevier Canada, a division of Reed Elsevier Canada, Ltd.

b. *Polyps*:

Mouth and pharynx

36. Define the following terms that relate to the oral cavity.

a. *Leukoplakia*:

b. *Varicosities*:

c. *Exostosis*:

Pharynx

Perform an examination of pharyngeal structures to rule out infection, inflammation, or lesions.

Neck

37. Assessment of the neck includes ______, ______, ______, ______, ______, and ______.

Thorax and Lungs

Posterior thorax

38. Define *vocal or tactile fremitus.*

39. Define the following normal breath sounds heard over the posterior thorax.

a. *Vesicular*:

b. *Bronchovesicular*:

c. *Bronchial:*

40. Complete the following table of adventitious breath sounds.

Sounds	Site Auscultated	Cause	Character
Crackles			
Rhonchi (sonorous wheeze)			
Wheezes (sibilant wheeze)			
Pleural friction rub			

Anterior thorax

Inspect the anterior thorax for the same features as the posterior thorax.

Heart

41. Explain the following terms related to assessment of the heart.

a. *Point of maximal impulse*:

b. S_1:

c. S_2:

d. S_3:

e. S_4:

Copyright © 2019 Elsevier Canada, a division of Reed Elsevier Canada, Ltd.

Inspection and palpation

42. Identify the appropriate sites for inspection and palpation of the following:

a. Angle of Louis:

b. Aortic area:

c. Pulmonic area:

d. Second pulmonic area:

e. Tricuspid area:

f. Mitral area:

g. Epigastric area:

Auscultation

43. Auscultation of the heart detects normal ______ ______, ______, and ______ ______.

44. Define *murmur.*

45. List the six factors to assess when a murmur is detected.

a. ______
b. ______
c. ______
d. ______
e. ______
f. ______

Vascular System

46. Explain the following conditions that are related to the vascular system.

a. *Syncope*:

b. *Occlusion*:

c. *Atherosclerosis*:

d. *Bruit*:

Jugular veins

47. Explain the steps the nurse would use to assess venous pressure.

a. ______
b. ______
c. ______
d. ______
e. ______

Peripheral arteries and veins

48. Complete the following table by listing the signs of venous and arterial insufficiency.

Assessment Criterion	Venous	Arterial
Colour		
Temperature		
Pulse		
Edema		
Skin changes		

Copyright © 2019 Elsevier Canada, a division of Reed Elsevier Canada, Ltd.

49. Describe how you would assess for *phlebitis.*

Breasts

50. The Canadian Cancer Society Steering Committee (2016) recommends the following for the early detection of breast cancer:

Palpation

51. Define the following terms.

a. *Metastasize*:

b. *Benign (fibrocystic) breast disease:*

Abdomen

52. Define the following terms related to the abdomen.

a. *Striae*:

b. *Hernias:*

c. *Distension*:

d. *Peristalsis:*

e. *Paralytic ileus:*

f. *Borborygmi:*

g. *Rebound tenderness*:

h. *Aneurysm*:

Female Genitalia and Reproductive Tract

53. Describe the following terms related to the female genitourinary tract.

a. *Chancres:*

b. *Papanicolaou (Pap) smear:*

Male Genitalia

54. Identify the common symptoms of testicular cancer.

Rectum and Anus

55. The purpose of the digital examination is:

Musculoskeletal System

General inspection

56. Define the following terms.

a. *Kyphosis:*

b. *Lordosis*:

Copyright © 2019 Elsevier Canada, a division of Reed Elsevier Canada, Ltd.

c. *Scoliosis:*

d. *Osteoporosis:*

Muscle tone and strength

57. Identify the correct range of motion for the following terms.

a. *Flexion:*

b. *Extension:*

c. *Hyperextension:*

d. *Pronation:*

e. *Supination:*

f. *Abduction:*

g. *Adduction:*

h. *Internal rotation:*

i. *External rotation:*

j. *Eversion:*

k. *Inversion:*

l. *Dorsiflexion:*

m. *Plantar flexion:*

58. Define the following terms related to muscle tone and strength.

a. *Hypertonicity:*

b. *Hypotonicity:*

c. *Atrophy:*

Neurologic System

Mental and emotional status

59. The purpose of the Mini-Mental State Examination is to measure ______ and ______.

60. Delirium is characterized by ______, ______, and ______.

61. The purpose of the Glasgow Coma Scale is to ______.

62. Briefly explain the two types of aphasia.

a. *Receptive:*

b. *Expressive:*

Intellectual function

Intellectual function includes memory, knowledge, abstract thinking, association, and judgement.

Cranial nerve function

63. Identify the 12 cranial nerves.

a.

b.

c.

d.

e.

f.

g.

h.

i.

j.

k.

l.

Sensory function

64. The sensory pathways of the central nervous system conduct what type of sensations?

Copyright © 2019 Elsevier Canada, a division of Reed Elsevier Canada, Ltd.

65. Identify how to assess sensory nerve function.

______

______

Motor function

66. Identify the functions of the cerebellum.

______

______

Reflexes

67. Identify the two types of normal reflexes.

a. ______

b. ______

REVIEW QUESTIONS

Select the appropriate answer, and cite the rationale for choosing that particular answer.

1. Which component should receive the highest priority before a physical examination?
   a. Preparation of the equipment
   b. Preparation of the environment
   c. Physical preparation of the patient
   d. Psychologic preparation of the patient

Answer: ______ Rationale: ______

2. Which method should the nurse use when assessing skin turgor of the patient?
   a. Inspecting the buccal mucosa with a penlight
   b. Palpating the skin with the dorsum of the hand
   c. Grasping a fold of skin on the back of the forearm and releasing
   d. Pressing the skin for 5 seconds, releasing, and noting each centimetre of depth

Answer: ______ Rationale: ______

3. While examining Mr. Polanzky, the nurse notes a circumscribed elevation of skin filled with serous fluid on his upper lip. The lesion is 0.4 cm in diameter. Which type of lesion is noted by the nurse?
   a. Macule
   b. Nodule
   c. Vesicle
   d. Pustule

Answer: ______ Rationale: ______

4. What is the proper technique used when assessing a patient's thorax?
   a. Complete the left side and then the right side
   b. Compare symmetrical areas from side to side
   c. Begin with the posterior lobes on the right side
   d. Change the position of the stethoscope between inspiration and expiration

Answer: ______ Rationale: ______

5. In a patient with pneumonia, the nurse hears high-pitched, continuous musical sounds over the bronchi and bronchioles that become louder on expiration. What sounds are described?
   a. Rhonchi
   b. Crackles
   c. Wheezes
   d. Friction rubs

Answer: ______ Rationale: ______

6. When auscultating heart sounds, what best describes the first heart sound (S_1)?
   a. Systole begins.
   b. There is rapid ventricular filling.
   c. The mitral and tricuspid valves close.
   d. The aortic and pulmonic valves close.

Answer: ______ Rationale: ______

Copyright © 2019 Elsevier Canada, a division of Reed Elsevier Canada, Ltd.

33 Infection Control

PRELIMINARY READING

Chapter 33, pages 683–726

COMPREHENSIVE UNDERSTANDING

Practices or techniques that control or prevent transmission of infection help to create an environment that protects patients and health care workers from disease.

Scientific Knowledge Base

1. An infection is ____.

2. Define the term *communicable.*

____

Chain of infection

3. Development of an infection occurs in a cycle that depends on the following elements.
   a. ______________________
   b. ______________________
   c. ______________________
   d. ______________________
   e. ______________________
   f. ______________________

Infectious Agents

4. Microorganisms include ______________, ______________, ______________, and ______________.

5. Define the following terms.
   a. *Virulence:*
   b. *Immunocompromised:*

6. The potential for microorganisms to cause disease depends on four factors. Name them.
   a. ______________________
   b. ______________________
   c. ______________________
   d. ______________________

Reservoir

7. Define *reservoir.*

8. Define *carriers.*

9. To thrive, organisms require the following. Briefly explain each one.
   a. Food:
   b. Oxygen (or lack of oxygen):
   c. Water:
   d. Temperature:
   e. pH:
   f. Minimal light:

Copyright © 2019 Elsevier Canada, a division of Reed Elsevier Canada, Ltd.

Portal of Exit

10. What is a portal of exit? Give examples.

____
____
____
____

Modes of Transmission

11. List the major modes of transmission of microorganisms from the reservoir to the host.

____
____
____
____

Portal of Entry

Organisms can enter the body through the same routes they use to exit.

Susceptible Host

12. Explain *susceptibility.*

____
____

The infectious process

13. The severity of the patient's illness depends on the ____________________, the ____________________, and the ____________________.

14. Describe the two types of infections.

a. *Localized:*

____
____

b. *Systemic:*

____
____

Defences against infection

15. The immune response is ____________________.

16. Explain the normal body's defences against infection.

a. Normal flora:

____
____
____

b. Body system defences:

____
____
____

c. Inflammation:

____
____
____

17. For each body system or organ in the grid that follows, identify at least one defence mechanism and the primary action to prevent infection.

System/Organ	Defence Mechanism	Action
Skin		
Mouth		
Eye		
Respiratory tract		
Urinary tract		
Gastrointestinal tract		
Vagina		

18. The *inflammatory response* includes the following. Explain each briefly.

a. Vascular and cellular responses:

____
____
____

b. Inflammatory exudates:

____
____
____

Copyright © 2019 Elsevier Canada, a division of Reed Elsevier Canada, Ltd.

c. Tissue repair:

19. Briefly explain the following vascular and cellular responses.

a. *Edema:*

b. *Phagocytosis:*

Health care–associated infections

20. Define *health care–associated infection (HAI) or nosocomial infection.*

21. Define the following types of HAIs.

a. *Exogenous:*

b. *Endogenous:*

22. Identify at least three factors that increase a hospitalized patient's risk of acquiring a HAI.

a.

b.

c.

23. Identify the major sites for nosocomial infection (HAI).

Nursing Process in Infection Control

Assessment

Nurses assess the patient's defence mechanisms, susceptibility, and knowledge of infections.

Knowing the factors that increase the patient's susceptibility or risk for infection, you are better able to plan preventive therapy that includes aseptic technique.

Status of defence mechanisms

You can determine the status of the patient's normal defence mechanisms against infection through a review of the physical assessment findings and the patient's medical condition.

24. Any reduction in the body's primary or secondary defences against infection places a patient at risk. List at least four risk factors of each.

a. Inadequate primary defences:

b. Inadequate secondary defences:

Patient susceptibility

25. The following factors influence patient susceptibility to infection. Explain each one.

a. Age:

b. Nutritional status:

c. Stress:

d. Disease process:

e. Medical therapy:

Clinical appearance

26. Describe the signs and symptoms of each type of infection.

a. Localized infection:

Copyright © 2019 Elsevier Canada, a division of Reed Elsevier Canada, Ltd.

b. Systemic infection:

____

____

____

27. Describe how an infection is manifested in an older person.

____

____

____

____

Laboratory data

28. List at least five laboratory values that may indicate infection.

a. ______________________________
b. ______________________________
c. ______________________________
d. ______________________________
e. ______________________________

Patient with infection

29. The ways in which infection can affect the patient's and family's needs may be ______________, ______________, ______________, or ______________.

Nursing Diagnosis

You may diagnose a risk for infection or make diagnoses that result from the effects of infection on health status.

Planning

Goals and outcomes

30. List four common goals of care relating to infection.

a. ______________________________
b. ______________________________
c. ______________________________
d. ______________________________

IMPLEMENTATION

Health promotion

31. List five ways you may prevent an infection from developing or spreading.

a. ______________________________
b. ______________________________
c. ______________________________
d. ______________________________
e. ______________________________

32. List preventive interventions to protect a patient from invasion by pathogens.

____

____

____

____

Acute care measures

Treatment of an infectious process includes eliminating the infectious organisms and supporting the patient's defences.

Asepsis

33. Define the following terms.

a. *Asepsis:*

____

____

b. *Medical asepsis:*

____

____

You are responsible for providing the patient with a safe environment. Your failure to be meticulous places the patient at risk for an infection that can seriously impair recovery or lead to death.

Control or Elimination of Infectious Agents

34. Explain the following methods of controlling or eliminating infectious agents.

a. Cleaning:

____

____

____

b. Disinfection:

____

____

____

c. Sterilization:

____

____

____

d. Control or elimination of reservoirs:

____

____

____

e. Control of portals of exit:

____

____

____

Copyright © 2019 Elsevier Canada, a division of Reed Elsevier Canada, Ltd.

f. Control of transmission:

g. Hand hygiene:

35. Describe the Centers for Disease Control and Prevention (CDC) guidelines on handwashing and the use of alcohol-based waterless antiseptics.

a.
b.
c.
d.
e.
f.
g.
h.
i.

Control of Portals of Entry

36. Many measures that control the exit of microorganisms also control the entrance of pathogens. Give at least five examples.

a.
b.
c.
d.
e.

Protection of the Susceptible Host

37. A patient's resistance to infection improves as the nurse protects the body's normal defences against infection. Explain.

Isolation Guidelines

38. Standard precautions or routine practices call for the appropriate use of protective devices and clothing, including ______, ______, ______, and ______.

39. Barrier protection is indicated for use with all patients because every patient has the potential to ______.

40. The CDC's (1996) and Health Canada's (1999) isolation guidelines contain a two-tiered approach. Explain.

a. Routine practices (first tier):

b. Isolation precautions (second tier):

41. List four basic principles common to all categories of isolation precautions.

a.
b.
c.
d.

Psychologic Implications of Isolation Precautions.

42. Briefly summarize the psychologic implications of isolation.

Specimen Collection.

43. Explain the techniques for collecting specimens from the patient with a suspected infection.

a. Wound:

b. Blood:

c. Stool:

Copyright © 2019 Elsevier Canada, a division of Reed Elsevier Canada, Ltd.

d. Urine: ______________________

____

Bagging Waste or Linen.

44. Explain Health Canada's recommendations for bagging waste or linen.

____

Transporting Patients.

45. Describe how you would transport a patient with an infection.

____

Role of the Infection Control Professional

46. List eight responsibilities of the infection control professional.

a. ______________________
b. ______________________
c. ______________________
d. ______________________
e. ______________________
f. ______________________
g. ______________________
h. ______________________

Patient Education

47. List six topics you need to discuss with the patient in relation to infection control practices.

a. ______________________
b. ______________________
c. ______________________
d. ______________________
e. ______________________
f. ______________________

Surgical Asepsis

48. Briefly explain what is meant by the concepts of *surgical asepsis* and *medical asepsis*.

____

49. Explain when surgical asepsis must be used.

____

Patient Preparation.

50. List three teaching points that reduce the risk of patient-associated contamination during sterile procedures or treatments.

a. ______________________
b. ______________________
c. ______________________

Principles of Surgical Asepsis.

51. List the seven principles of surgical asepsis.

a. ______________________
b. ______________________
c. ______________________
d. ______________________
e. ______________________
f. ______________________
g. ______________________

Performing Sterile Procedures.

52. List and briefly explain the nine steps in the preparation of a sterile field.

a. ______________________
b. ______________________
c. ______________________
d. ______________________
e. ______________________
f. ______________________
g. ______________________
h. ______________________
i. ______________________

Copyright © 2019 Elsevier Canada, a division of Reed Elsevier Canada, Ltd.

Evaluation

The success of infection control techniques is measured by determining whether the goals for reducing or preventing infection are achieved.

Two important skills in evaluation are the ability to correctly assess wounds for healing and the ability to conduct a physical assessment of body systems.

A clear description of any signs and symptoms of systemic or local infection is necessary to give all nurses a baseline for comparative evaluation.

The patient at risk for infection must understand the measures needed to reduce or prevent microorganism growth and spread.

REVIEW QUESTIONS

Select the appropriate answer, and cite the rationale for choosing that particular answer.

1. Which of the following is *not* an element in the chain of infection?
   a. Infectious agent or pathogen
   b. Reservoir for pathogen growth
   c. Mode of transmission
   d. Formation of immunoglobulin

Answer:______________ Rationale:______________

____

____

2. Which of the following is *not* a *pathogenic* organism?
   a. Bacteria
   b. Leukocyte
   c. Virus
   d. Fungus

Answer:______________ Rationale:______________

____

____

3. When considering the severity of a patient's illness, what will it *not* depend on?
   a. Extent of infection
   b. Pathogenicity of the microorganism
   c. Susceptibility of the host
   d. Incubation period

Answer:______________ Rationale:______________

____

____

4. Which of the following best describes an iatrogenic infection or HAI?
   a. It results from a diagnostic or therapeutic procedure.
   b. It occurs when patients are infected with their own organisms as a result of immunodeficiency.
   c. It involves an incubation period of 3 to 4 weeks before it can be detected.
   d. It results from an extended infection of the urinary tract.

Answer:______________ Rationale:______________

____

____

5. Which of the following best describes a field contamination when the nurse is setting up a sterile field on the patient's over-bed table?
   a. The nurse keeps the top of the table above his or her waist.
   b. Sterile saline solution is spilled on the field.
   c. Sterile objects are kept within a 2.5-cm border of the field.
   d. The nurse, who has a cold, wears a double mask.

Answer:______________ Rationale:______________

____

____

6. When airborne or droplet isolation precautions are being observed for a patient who must be transported to another part of the hospital, which of the following is *not* required of you as the nurse?
   a. Place a mask on the patient before leaving the room.
   b. Obtain a physician's order to prohibit the patient from being transported.
   c. Advise personnel in diagnostic or procedural areas that the patient is under isolation precautions.
   d. Provide the patient with tissues and a bag for proper disposal of secretions.

Answer:______________ Rationale:______________

____

____

Copyright © 2019 Elsevier Canada, a division of Reed Elsevier Canada, Ltd.

34 Medication Administration

PRELIMINARY READING

Chapter 34, pages 727–814

COMPREHENSIVE UNDERSTANDING

A medication is a substance used in the prevention, diagnosis, relief, treatment, or cure of health alterations.

Scientific Knowledge Base

Medication administration and evaluation are essential to nursing practice; you need to understand the actions and effects of the medications your patients take.

Pharmacologic concepts

Drug Names

1. A single medication may have three different names. Define each one.

   a. Chemical name:

   ____

   ____

   b. Generic name:

   ____

   ____

   c. Trade name:

   ____

   ____

Classification

2. A medication classification indicates

   ______________________________.

Medication Forms

3. The form of the medication determines its ________

   ______________________________.

Medication legislation and standards

Canadian Drug Legislation

4. Briefly summarize the role of the federal government in medication regulation.

   ____

   ____

   ____

   ____

Drug Standards

5. Official publications set standards for medications in the following areas.

   a. ______________________________

   b. ______________________________

   c. ______________________________

   d. ______________________________

   e. ______________________________

   f. ______________________________

Control

6. The Health Protection Branch (HPB) is responsible

   for ______________________________.

Provincial, Territorial, and Local Regulation of Medications

7. Summarize the role of the provincial government in medication regulation.

   ____

   ____

   ____

   ____

8. Summarize the role of health care institutions with regard to government medication regulation.

   ____

   ____

   ____

   ____

Medication Regulation and Nursing Practice

9. Describe why it is important for registered nurses to be aware of both federal and provincial regulations affecting medication administration in their practice.

   ____

   ____

   ____

   ____

Copyright © 2019 Elsevier Canada, a division of Reed Elsevier Canada, Ltd.

Pharmacokinetics as the basis of medication actions

10. *Pharmacokinetics* is the study of

_______________________________________.

Absorption

11. Define *absorption.*

12. Briefly explain the following factors that influence drug absorption.

    a. Route of administration:

    b. Ability of a medication to dissolve:

    c. Blood flow to the site of administration:

    d. Body surface area:

    e. Lipid solubility of a medication:

Before administering any medication, check pharmacology books, drug references, or package inserts, or consult with pharmacists to identify medication–medication interactions or medication–nutrient interactions.

Distribution

The rate and extent of distribution depend on the physical and chemical properties of the medication and on the physiology of the person taking the medication.

13. Explain how each of the following affect the rate and extent of medication distribution.

    a. Circulation:

    b. Membrane permeability:

    c. Protein binding:

Metabolism

14. Define *biotransformation*, and identify where it occurs.

15. Explain why biotransformation is an important concept for registered nurses to understand.

Excretion

16. After drugs are metabolized, they exit the body through the following routes:

17. Identify the primary organ for medication excretion, and explain what happens if this organ's function declines.

Types of medication action

Medications vary considerably in the way they act and in their types of action. Factors other than characteristics of the medication also influence medication actions. A patient does not always respond in the same way to each successive dose of a medication, and the same medication causes very different responses in different patients.

18. Define the following predicted or unintended effects of medications, and provide a nursing practice example.

    a. Therapeutic effects:

    b. Side effects:

Copyright © 2019 Elsevier Canada, a division of Reed Elsevier Canada, Ltd.

c. Adverse effects:

d. Toxic effects:

e. Idiosyncratic reactions:

f. Allergic reactions:

g. Anaphylactic reactions:

Medication interactions

19. Describe the process of a medication–medication interaction, and provide an example from nursing practice.

20. Describe the concept of a *synergistic effect*, and provide an example from nursing practice.

Medication dose responses

When a medication is prescribed, the goal is to achieve a constant blood level within a safe therapeutic range.

Repeated doses are required to achieve a constant therapeutic concentration of a medication because a portion of a drug is always being excreted.

21. Define the following terms.

a. *Serum concentration:*

b. *Serum half-life:*

22. Using the concepts of serum concentration and serum half-life, explain why it is important for both patients and nurses to follow regular dosage schedules and adhere to prescribed doses and dose intervals.

23. Explain the following time intervals of medication actions.

a. Onset of drug action:

b. Peak:

c. Trough:

d. Duration of action:

e. Plateau:

Routes of administration

The route prescribed for a medication's administration depends on its properties, the desired effect, and the patient's physical and mental condition.

Oral Routes

The oral route is the easiest and the most commonly used route.

24. Identify the types of oral routes, explain how the oral routes are used, and identify the effects of using these routes.

Copyright © 2019 Elsevier Canada, a division of Reed Elsevier Canada, Ltd.

Parenteral Routes

The parenteral route involves administering a drug through injection into body tissues.

25. List the four major sites of parenteral injections.
    a. ______
    b. ______
    c. ______
    d. ______

26. Define the following advanced techniques of medication administration.
    a. Epidural:
    ______
    ______
    b. Intrathecal:
    ______
    ______
    c. Intraosseous:
    ______
    ______
    d. Intraperitoneal:
    ______
    ______
    e. Intrapleural:
    ______
    ______
    f. Intraarterial:
    ______
    ______
    g. Intracardiac:
    ______
    ______
    h. Intraarticular:
    ______
    ______

Topical Administration

Medications that are applied to the skin and mucous membranes generally have local effects.

27. Identify five methods for applying medications to mucous membranes.
    a. ______
    b. ______
    c. ______
    d. ______
    e. ______

Inhalation Route

Medications that are administered by the inhalation route are readily absorbed and work rapidly. Inhaled medications may have either local or systemic effects.

28. Describe the three passages through which *inhalations* can be administered.
    a. Nasal:
    ______
    ______
    b. Oral:
    ______
    ______
    c. Endotracheal or tracheal:
    ______
    ______

Intraocular Route

29. Describe the process of *intraocular medication delivery*.
    ______
    ______
    ______
    ______

Systems of medication measurement

The proper administration of a medication depends on your ability to compute medication doses accurately and to measure medications correctly. Mistakes can lead to a fatal error.

30. The following are measuring systems used in medication therapy. Briefly explain their basic units.
    a. *Metric system:*
    ______
    ______
    b. *Household measurements:*
    ______
    ______

31. A solution is ______
    ______.

Copyright © 2019 Elsevier Canada, a division of Reed Elsevier Canada, Ltd.

Nursing Knowledge Base

More people die from medical errors than from motor vehicle accidents, breast cancer, and workplace injuries.

32. To safely administer medications, ensure that you know __________, __________, and __________.

Clinical calculations

To administer medications safely, you need an understanding of basic arithmetic to calculate medication doses, mix solutions, and perform a variety of other activities. This skill is important because medications are not always dispensed in the unit of measure in which they are ordered.

Household Measurements

34. Complete the following measurement equivalents.

Metric	Household
1 mL	___drops
___mL	1 tablespoon
30 mL	___tablespoon(s)
___mL	1 cup
___mL	1 pint
___mL	1 quart

35. Complete the following conversions.

a. 100 mg = __________ g

b. 2.5 L = __________ mL

c. 500 mL = __________ L

d. 15 mg = __________ g

e. 30 gtt = __________ mL

f. 1/6 g = __________ mg

Dose Calculations

36. Write out the formula used to determine the correct dose when preparing solid or liquid forms of medications.

____

37. Define the following terms.

a. *Dose ordered:*

____

____

b. *Dose on hand:*

____

____

Conversions Within One System

33. Indicate which direction the decimal point is moved for the following mathematical calculations in the metric system, and provide a rationale.

a. Division:

____

____

b. Multiplication:

____

____

c. *Amount on hand:*

____

____

38. If half a tablet is required, then have __________ prepare and send the proper dose, as even a __________ tablet can lead to medication errors.

Liquid medications are often manufactured in volumes greater than 1 mL. In applying the formula, be careful to use the correct concentration to avoid a medication error.

Pediatric Doses

39. Write out the formula applied to accurately calculate safe pediatric doses.

____

____

40. Explain why calculating children's medication doses requires caution.

____

____

____

____

Copyright © 2019 Elsevier Canada, a division of Reed Elsevier Canada, Ltd.

41. The nurse who is administering the medications is accountable for

____

_______________.

Prescriber's role

42. Identify the primary responsibilities of the prescriber in giving medications to patients.

____

43. Identify recommendations to reduce medication errors associated with both verbal medication orders and prescriptions.

____

44. Use caution when you use abbreviations because some _______________ can lead to _______________ and the potential for _______________.

Types of orders

45. Briefly explain the five common types of medication orders.

a. Routine medication orders:

b. As needed ("prn") orders:

c. Single (one-time) orders:

d. STAT orders:

e. Now orders:

Prescriptions

46. List the six parts of a prescription.

a. _______________
b. _______________
c. _______________
d. _______________
e. _______________
f. _______________

Pharmacist's role

47. Identify the primary responsibility of the pharmacist in the administration of medications.

____

Distribution systems

48. List the three medication distribution systems, and identify the advantages and disadvantages of each.

a. _______________

b. _______________

c. _______________

Nurse's role

49. Summarize the nurse's primary responsibilities when administering medications, and explain why these responsibilities are important in nursing practice.

____

50. A medication error is

_______________.

51. Identify steps that registered nurses can take to prevent medication errors.

____

Copyright © 2019 Elsevier Canada, a division of Reed Elsevier Canada, Ltd.

52. Explain what steps you should take if a medication error occurs.
    a. ______
    b. ______
    c. ______
    d. ______

53. Identify sources of medication errors.
    a. ______
    b. ______
    c. ______
    d. ______
    e. ______
    f. ______
    g. ______
    h. ______
    i. ______

54. Briefly describe *medication reconciliation.*

______

______

______

Critical Thinking

Knowledge

55. Summarize the knowledge needed from other disciplines to safely administer medications.

______

______

______

______

Experience

Psychomotor skills, the patient's attitudes, knowledge, physical and mental status, and responses can make medication administration a complex experience.

Cognitive and behavioural attributes

56. Demonstrating accountability and responsibility when administering medications means that the nurse ______.

Standards

57. List the "10 rights" of medication administration, and briefly explain each one.
    a. ______
    b. ______
    c. ______
    d. ______
    e. ______
    f. ______
    g. ______
    h. ______
    i. ______
    j. ______

58. Explain the importance of adhering to agency policies and procedures when administering medications.

______

______

______

______

Maintaining Patients' Rights

59. Because of the potential risks related to medication administration, patients have the right to the following:
    a. ______
    b. ______
    c. ______
    d. ______
    e. ______
    f. ______
    g. ______
    h. ______

Nursing Process and Medication Administration

Assessment

60. Describe the following elements of nursing assessment, and explain each element's significance as related to safe medication administration.
    a. History:
    ______
    ______
    b. History of allergies:
    ______
    ______
    c. Medication data:
    ______
    ______
    d. Diet history:
    ______
    ______
    e. Patient's perceptual or coordination problems:
    ______
    ______

Copyright © 2019 Elsevier Canada, a division of Reed Elsevier Canada, Ltd.

f. Patient's current condition:

g. Patient's attitude toward medication use:

h. Patient's knowledge and understanding of medication therapy:

i. Patient's learning needs:

Nursing Diagnosis

Assessment provides data on the patient's condition, ability to self-administer medications, and medication use patterns. This information can be used to determine actual or potential problems with medication therapy.

61. Identify potential nursing diagnoses that apply to the process of medication administration.

Planning

Organize nursing care activities to ensure the safe administration of medications.

Goals and outcomes

62. Identify a goal and related outcomes that the nurse or patient needs to meet before the administration of medications, and provide the rationale for each goal and outcome.

Setting priorities

Prioritize care when administering medications. Use information gathered from your assessment of the patient to determine whether the administration of medications is appropriate and, if it is, which medication should be given first.

Implementation

Health promotion

63. Identify factors that can influence the patient's compliance with the medication regimen, and provide the rationale for your answers.

64. Identify important information that you should provide to the patient and family in relation to medications, and provide the rationale for your answers.

Acute care

65. Identify the necessary components of medication orders.

66. Explain why the following interventions are essential for safe and effective medication administration.

a. Receiving medication orders:

b. Correct transcription and communication of orders:

c. Accurate dose calculation and measurement:

d. Correct administration:

e. Recording medication administration:

Copyright © 2019 Elsevier Canada, a division of Reed Elsevier Canada, Ltd.

Restorative care

67. Regardless of the type of medication activity, you are responsible for ______________________.

Special considerations for administering medications to specific age groups

Infants and Children

68. Identify strategies to address children's psychosocial preparation before administering medications.

____

____

____

____

Older Persons

69. Identify special considerations for older persons when administering medication, and provide rationales.

____

____

____

____

Polypharmacy

70. *Polypharmacy* occurs when ______________, ______________, ______________, or ______________.

71. Describe the difference between *rational polypharmacy* and *irrational polypharmacy*.

____

____

____

____

Noncompliance

72. Noncompliance is defined as a ______________ of medication, such as ______________ a prescribed medication or ______________ the dose of a medication.

Evaluation

You must know the therapeutic action and common side effects of each medication to monitor a patient's response to that medication.

73. Many different evaluation measures can be used in the context of medication administration. Identify various measures used in practice to evaluate medication administration processes.

____

____

____

____

74. The most common type of measurement used to evaluate medication administration is ______________ ______________________.

Medication Administration

Oral administration

The easiest and most desirable way to administer medications is by mouth.

75. The primary contraindications to giving oral medications include ______________________.

76. To protect the patient against possible aspiration, what nursing assessments should be conducted? What nursing interventions should be implemented? Provide rationales for your answers.

____

____

____

____

Topical medication applications

Topical medications are applied locally, most often to intact skin. They can also be applied to mucous membranes.

Skin Applications

Many locally applied medications, such as lotions, pastes, and ointments, cause both systemic and local effects; apply these medications using gloves and applicators.

77. Explain the procedure for administering the following skin applications.

    a. Ointment:

    ____

    ____

    b. Lotion:

    ____

    ____

    c. Transdermal patch:

    ____

    ____

Copyright © 2019 Elsevier Canada, a division of Reed Elsevier Canada, Ltd.

Nasal Instillation

78. Summarize the rationale for nasal instillations.

Eye Instillation

79. List four principles for administering eye instillations.

 a. ______
 b. ______
 c. ______
 d. ______

Intraocular Administration

80. Summarize the procedure for administering ophthalmic medications, and provide rationales for steps specific to ophthalmic medication delivery.

Ear Instillation

81. Explain the procedure for administering ear instillations.

 a. Adults:

 b. Children:

82. Identify the significant differences between adults and children when administering ear medications.

Vaginal Instillation

83. Vaginal medications are available as ______, ______, ______, and ______.

Rectal Instillation

84. Explain the differences between vaginal and rectal suppositories, and the reason for these differences.

85. Summarize the procedure for administering rectal suppositories, and provide rationales for steps specific to rectal suppository administration.

Administering medications by inhalation

86. Identify the most common conditions of patients who are prescribed medications via the inhalation route.

87. Summarize the procedure for teaching patients to self-administer medications via a metered-dose inhaler, and provide the rationale.

Administering medications by irrigations

88. Identify the principles you must adhere to when performing irrigations, and provide rationales for your answers.

Administering parenteral medications

When medications are administered parenterally, it is an invasive procedure that must be performed using aseptic techniques.

Each type of injection requires certain skills to ensure that the medication reaches the proper location.

Equipment

89. Identify the two major types of syringes.

 a. ______
 b. ______

Copyright © 2019 Elsevier Canada, a division of Reed Elsevier Canada, Ltd.

90. Identify three factors that must be considered when selecting a needle for an injection.
   a. ______
   b. ______
   c. ______

91. Identify the advantages of using the Tubex® or Carpuject® injection system.

______

Preparing an Injection from an Ampule

92. An ampule is a ______.

93. Summarize the procedure for withdrawing medication from an ampule, and provide the rationale for each step.

______

Preparing an Injection from a Vial

94. A vial is a ______.

The vial is a closed system, and air must be injected into it to permit easy withdrawal of the solution.

95. Summarize the procedure for withdrawing medication from a vial and provide a rationale for each step.

______

Mixing Medications

96. If two medications are compatible, it is possible to mix two drugs together into one injection if ______.

Mixing Medications from Two Vials

97. List the three principles to follow when mixing medications from two vials.
   a. ______
   b. ______
   c. ______

Mixing Medications from a Vial and an Ampule

98. When mixing medications from an ampule and a vial, which medication should be prepared first? Provide the rationale for your answer.

______

Insulin Preparation

99. Insulin is ______.

100. Explain why insulin must be administered by injection.

______

101. Insulin is classified by ______.

Insulin is ordered either by a specific dose at select times or by a sliding scale. A sliding scale dictates a certain dose on the basis of the patient's blood glucose level.

102. Summarize the procedure for mixing two kinds of insulin in the same syringe.

______

Administering injections

103. The characteristics of the tissues injected influence the ______.

104. List the techniques used to minimize patient discomfort associated with injections, and provide rationales for your answers.
   a. ______
   b. ______
   c. ______
   d. ______
   e. ______
   f. ______
   g. ______

Copyright © 2019 Elsevier Canada, a division of Reed Elsevier Canada, Ltd.

Subcutaneous Injections

Subcutaneous injections involve placing the medications into the loose connective tissue under the dermis.

105. Explain the differences in absorption between a subcutaneous and an intramuscular (IM) injection.

______

______

______

______

106. The best sites for subcutaneous injections include ______, ______, and ______.

107. The site chosen for a subcutaneous injection should be free of ______, ______, and ______.

108. Identify the maximum amount of water-soluble medication given by the subcutaneous route.

______

______

______

______

109. Identify the factors to consider when determining if a subcutaneous injection should be given at a 90- or 45-degree angle.

______

______

______

______

Intramuscular Injections

110. Identify some important things to consider when using the IM route.

______

______

______

______

111. The angle of insertion for an IM injection is ______ degrees.

112. Indicate the maximum volume of medication for IM injection in each of the following groups (provide rationales for your answers).

    a. Well-developed adult:

    ______

    ______

    b. Children, older persons, or thin persons:

    ______

    ______

    c. Older infants and small children:

    ______

    ______

    d. Smaller infants:

    ______

    ______

Sites

113. List the assessment criteria for selecting an IM site.

    a. ______

    b. ______

    c. ______

    d. ______

114. Describe the characteristics, advantages, and disadvantages of the following injection sites.

    a. Ventrogluteal:

    ______

    ______

    b. Vastus lateralis:

    ______

    ______

    c. Dorsogluteal:

    ______

    ______

    d. Deltoid:

    ______

    ______

Technique for IM Injections

115. Describe the Z-track technique for administering IM injections. Explain the rationale for using the *Z-track method* of injection.

______

______

______

______

Copyright © 2019 Elsevier Canada, a division of Reed Elsevier Canada, Ltd.

Intradermal Injections

116. Explain the rationale for using the intradermal route to administer medication.

Safety in Administering Medications by Injection

Needleless Devices

117. Explain the rationale for the use of a needleless device.

Intravenous Administration

118. The nurse administers medications intravenously by the following methods.

a. ______
b. ______
c. ______

119. Discuss the advantages of administering medications by the IV route.

Large-Volume Infusions

120. Identify the advantage and disadvantage of the large-volume infusion method (provide rationales for your answers).

Intravenous Bolus

121. Explain the advantage and disadvantage of the IV bolus route of administration (provide rationales for your answers).

Volume-Controlled Infusions

122. List the advantages of using volume-controlled infusions.

a. ______
b. ______
c. ______

Volume-Control Administration

123. Describe the setup and purpose of a volume-control administration set.

Piggyback

124. Describe the setup and purpose of a *piggyback set*.

Tandem

125. Describe the setup and purpose of a *tandem set*.

Mini-Infusion Pump

126. Describe the setup and purpose of a *mini-infusion pump*.

Intermittent Venous Access

127. List two advantages of using intermittent venous access devices.

a. ______
b. ______

Administration of IV Therapy in the Home

128. When receiving home IV therapy, patient education should include ______.

Copyright © 2019 Elsevier Canada, a division of Reed Elsevier Canada, Ltd.

Subcutaneous Butterfly Catheters

129. Briefly define *hypodermoclysis*, and list its advantages.

____

____

____

____

REVIEW QUESTIONS

Select the appropriate answer, and cite the rationale for choosing that particular answer.

1. Which term describes the study of how medications enter the body, reach their sites of action, are metabolized, and then exit from the body?
   a. Pharmacology
   b. Pharmacokinetics
   c. Pharmacopoeia
   d. Biopharmaceutica

Answer:______________ Rationale:______________

____

____

2. Which statement correctly characterizes medication absorption?
   a. Many medications must enter the systemic circulation to have a therapeutic effect.
   b. Mucous membranes are relatively impermeable to chemicals, making absorption slow.
   c. Oral medications are absorbed more quickly when administered with meals.
   d. Drugs administered subcutaneously are absorbed more quickly than those injected intramuscularly.

Answer:______________ Rationale:______________

____

____

3. When a drug is administered, which of the following best describes the *onset* of the medication?
   a. The time it takes for the medication to produce a response
   b. The time it takes for the medication to produce accelerated cellular process
   c. The time it takes for the medication to reach its highest effective concentration
   d. The time it takes for the medication to produce blood serum concentration and maintenance

Answer:______________ Rationale:______________

____

____

4. Which of the following is *not* a parenteral route of administration?
   a. Buccal
   b. Subcutaneous
   c. Intramuscular
   d. Intradermal

Answer:______________ Rationale:______________

____

____

5. Using the body surface area formula, what dose of drug X should a child who weighs 12 kg (body surface area = 0.54 m^2) receive if the normal adult dose of drug X is 300 mg?
   a. 50 mg
   b. 95 mg
   c. 100 mg
   d. 200 mg

Answer:______________ Rationale:______________

____

____

6. The nurse is preparing an insulin injection in which both short-acting (clear) and long-acting (cloudy) insulin will be mixed. Into which vial should the nurse inject air first?
   a. The vial of long-acting insulin
   b. The vial of short-acting insulin
   c. Either vial, as long as long-acting insulin is drawn up first
   d. Neither vial; it is not necessary to put air into vials before withdrawing medication

Answer:______________ Rationale:______________

____

____

Copyright © 2019 Elsevier Canada, a division of Reed Elsevier Canada, Ltd.

35 Complementary and Alternative Approaches in Health Care

PRELIMINARY READING

Chapter 35, pages 815–831

COMPREHENSIVE UNDERSTANDING

People desired a different kind of health care—one that embraced healing, acknowledgement of the spiritual dimensions of health and illness, and openness toward alternative medical systems.

Complementary, Alternative, and Integrative Approaches in Health Care

1. Describe the difference between the following terms.

   a. *Complementary approaches*:

   ____

   ____

   ____

   b. *Alternative approaches*:

   ____

   ____

   ____

2. Describe *integrative medicine.*

   ____

   ____

   ____

3. Complementary and alternative therapies are often organized into five categories that researchers find useful. List the five categories.

   a. ______________________________

   b. ______________________________

   c. ______________________________

   d. ______________________________

   e. ______________________________

4. Explain the following alternative therapies in the whole medical systems category and give an example of each.

   a. Ayurveda:

   ____

   ____

   ____

   b. Latin American practices:

   ____

   ____

   ____

   c. Traditional Indigenous medicine:

   ____

   ____

   ____

   d. Naturopathic medicine:

   ____

   ____

   ____

   e. Traditional Chinese medicine (TCM):

   ____

   ____

   ____

Public interest in complementary and alternative medicine approaches

5. Describe *integrative medicine programs.*

   ____

   ____

   ____

   ____

In Canada and worldwide, demand is growing for alternative medicines and the services of alternative health care providers. The persons who use complementary and alternative medicine (CAM) therapies typically are women with a post–high school or college-equivalent education.

Complementary and alternative medicine therapies and holistic nursing

The practice of holistic nursing regards and treats the patient's mind, body, and spirit. Holistic interventions can augment standard treatments, replace ineffective or debilitating interventions, and promote and maintain health.

Copyright © 2019 Elsevier Canada, a division of Reed Elsevier Canada, Ltd.

6. Discuss the two types of CAM therapies.
   a. ______
   b. ______

Nursing-Accessible Approaches

Some CAM therapies and techniques use natural processes, such as breathing, concentration, and simple touch, to help patients feel better and cope with their chronic conditions.

7. CAM therapies should be chosen ______.

Relaxation therapy

8. Define the *stress response.*

______

9. *Relaxation* is ______.

10. *Progressive relaxation* training helps to ______.

11. *Passive relaxation* involves teaching ______.

Clinical Applications of Relaxation Therapy

12. Relaxation techniques can lower ______, decrease ______, improve ______, and reduce ______.

13. The type of relaxation intervention should be matched to ______.

Limitations of Relaxation Therapy

14. Identify the limitations of relaxation therapy.

______

Meditation and breathing

15. *Meditation* is ______.

Clinical Applications of Meditation

16. Identify the clinical applications of meditation.

______

Imagery

17. *Imagery* (visualization techniques) is ______.

Clinical applications of imagery

18. Identify the clinical applications of imagery.

______

Training-Specific Therapies

Biofeedback

19. *Biofeedback* is ______.

Clinical Applications of Biofeedback

20. Identify the clinical applications of biofeedback.

______

Therapeutic touch

21. *Therapeutic touch (TT)* is ______.

Clinical Applications of Therapeutic Touch

22. Identify the clinical applications of TT and healing touch.

______

Chiropractic medicine

23. *Chiropractic medicine* is ______.

Clinical Applications of Chiropractic Medicine

24. Describe the clinical applications of chiropractic medicine.

______

Traditional chinese medicine

25. TCM blends several healing modalities, including ______, with scientific principles.

Copyright © 2019 Elsevier Canada, a division of Reed Elsevier Canada, Ltd.

26. Explain the concept of *yin and yang.*

27. *Qi* is ________________.

28. Another important component of Chinese medicine involves five elements; list them below.

a.
b.
c.
d.
e.

29. Define *meridians.*

Acupuncture

30. *Acupuncture* is ________________.

Clinical Applications of Acupuncture

31. Describe the clinical applications of acupuncture.

Role of Nutrition in Disease Prevention and Health Promotion

Botanical therapies

32. The goal of *botanical therapy* is ________________.

33. Drug therapy is aimed at ________________.

Clinical applications of natural health products (NHPs)

34. Describe the clinical applications of botanical/natural health products.

35. Explain what a *natural product number (NPN)* is.

Limitations of NHPs

36. Identify the limitations of botanicals/natural health products.

Data does not support the use of these herbs in infants or children, or during pregnancy or lactation.

Nursing Role for Interprofessional Collaboration in CAM

37. Summarize the role of the nurse regarding CAM therapies.

REVIEW QUESTIONS

Select the appropriate answer, and cite the rationale for choosing that particular answer.

1. Why do patients choose to use unconventional therapies?
   a. They are willing to pay to feel better.
   b. Such therapies are now widely accepted by Health Canada's Office of Natural Health Products.
   c. They are dissatisfied with conventional medicine.
   d. They want religious approval for the remedies they use.

Answer:________________ Rationale:________________

2. Which herb is considered safe for the treatment of mild depression?
   a. Milk thistle
   b. St. John's wort
   c. Pokeroot
   d. Hawthorn

Answer:________________ Rationale:________________

Copyright © 2019 Elsevier Canada, a division of Reed Elsevier Canada, Ltd.

3. How can you best assess your patient's use of alternative therapies?
   a. Asking the patient true-or-false questions about his or her health
   b. Asking for a thorough medical history
   c. Reviewing laboratory studies that assess levels of certain herbs
   d. Asking open-ended questions on alternative therapies

Answer:_______________ Rationale:_______________

____

____

4. Which of the following steps should you take to be better informed about alternative therapies?
   a. Keep abreast of the current research on alternative therapies.
   b. Familiarize yourself with recent case studies on alternative therapies.
   c. Familiarize yourself with general principles of homeopathy.
   d. Review herb manufacturers' literature on specific herbs.

Answer:_______________ Rationale:_______________

____

____

Copyright © 2019 Elsevier Canada, a division of Reed Elsevier Canada, Ltd.

36 Activity and Exercise

PRELIMINARY READING

Chapter 36, pages 832–871

COMPREHENSIVE UNDERSTANDING

Body Alignment

1. Define *body alignment.*

____

____

____

____

Body Balance

2. *Body balance* is achieved when

______________________________.

3. Define *centre of gravity.*

____

____

____

____

4. Proper body alignment and posture are maintained by using the following two simple techniques.

   a. ______________________________

   b. ______________________________

Friction

5. Define *friction.*

____

____

____

6. List two techniques that minimize friction.

   a. ______________________________

   b. ______________________________

Physiology of movement

7. List three systems responsible for coordinating body movements.

   a. ______________________________

   b. ______________________________

   c. ______________________________

Skeletal System

8. List five functions of the skeletal system.

   a. ______________________________

   b. ______________________________

   c. ______________________________

   d. ______________________________

   e. ______________________________

9. Describe the following terms.

   a. *Joints*:

   ____

   ____

   b. *Synarthrotic joint*:

   ____

   ____

   c. *Cartilaginous joint*:

   ____

   ____

   d. *Fibrous joint*:

   ____

   ____

   e. *Synovial joint*:

   ____

   ____

Copyright © 2019 Elsevier Canada, a division of Reed Elsevier Canada, Ltd.

f. *Ligaments*:

g. *Tendons*:

h. *Cartilage*:

Skeletal Muscle

10. Briefly describe how skeletal muscles affect movement.

Muscles Concerned With Movement

11. Briefly explain the work of muscles concerned with *movement.*

Muscles Concerned With Posture

12. Briefly explain the work of muscles concerned with *posture.*

Muscle Groups

13. The nervous system regulates and coordinates the following different muscle groups. Briefly explain each.

a. *Antagonistic muscles*:

b. *Synergistic muscles*:

c. *Antigravity muscles*:

Skeletal muscles support posture and carry out voluntary movement. These muscles are attached to the skeleton by tendons, which provide strength and permit motion.

Nervous System

14. Briefly describe how movement and posture are regulated by the nervous system.

Proprioception

15. Define *proprioception.*

Balance

16. The structures in the ear that assist in maintaining balance are the ______.

Principles of body mechanics

17. List five principles of body mechanics.

a.
b.
c.
d.
e.

Pathologic influences on body mechanics and movement

18. Briefly explain how the following pathologic conditions may affect body alignment and mobility.

a. Congenital abnormalities:

b. Disorders of bones, joints, and muscles:

c. Central nervous system damage and disorders:

Copyright © 2019 Elsevier Canada, a division of Reed Elsevier Canada, Ltd.

d. Musculoskeletal trauma: ______

e. Other chronic diseases: ______

Exercise and activity

Exercise is physical activity for the purpose of conditioning the body, improving health, and maintaining fitness, or it may be used as a therapeutic measure.

Nursing Knowledge Base

Developmental changes

19. The greatest change and impact on the maturational process is observed ______.

20. Identify the descriptive characteristics of body alignment and mobility for the following age groups.

a. Infants through school-aged children: ______

b. Adolescents: ______

c. Young to middle-aged adults: ______

d. Older persons: ______

Behavioural aspects

21. Patients are more likely to incorporate an exercise program into their daily life if this choice is ______ and ______.

Environmental issues

22. Explain the exercise and activity issues related to the following sites.

a. Work sites: ______

b. Schools: ______

c. Community: ______

Cultural and ethnic influences

23. The nurse must consider what motivates and what is deemed appropriate and enjoyable when developing a physical fitness program for culturally diverse populations. Briefly describe a comprehensive fitness program that would be suitable for an ethnocultural group with which you interact.

______

Family and social support

24. Briefly explain how a family may be a motivational tool in regard to physical fitness.

______

Nursing Process

Assessment

Body alignment

25. Briefly explain how the assessment of body alignment and posture is carried out.

______

Mobility

26. There are several components to assess in regard to mobility. Explain each.

a. *Range of motion (ROM)*: ______

Copyright © 2019 Elsevier Canada, a division of Reed Elsevier Canada, Ltd.

b. *Gait*:

____

____

c. *Exercise and activity*:

____

____

Activity Tolerance

27. Identify three factors that affect activity tolerance.

a. ______________________________

b. ______________________________

c. ______________________________

Nursing Diagnosis

28. Assessment of the patient's ____________, ____________, ____________, and ____________ provides clusters of data or defining characteristics that can lead you to a nursing diagnosis.

29. Give five examples of nursing diagnoses related to exercise and activity.

a. ______________________________

b. ______________________________

c. ______________________________

d. ______________________________

e. ______________________________

Planning

30. The plan should include consideration of the following:

a. ______________________________

b. ______________________________

c. ______________________________

d. ______________________________

e. ______________________________

Implementation

Health promotion

31. List the three recommendations for adult exercise.

a. ______________________________

b. ______________________________

c. ______________________________

32. Explain how to calculate the patient's maximum heart rate.

____

____

____

____

33. An exercise program should include the following aspects. Explain each.

a. Aerobic exercise:

____

____

b. Stretching and flexibility exercises:

____

____

c. Resistance training:

____

____

Acute care

Patients in acute care often have reduced activity tolerance or are immobile to varying degrees. Promoting activity and preventing the effects of immobility are paramount.

The musculoskeletal system can be maintained by encouraging the use of stretching and isometric-type exercises.

34. Briefly explain the technique of *isometric exercises*.

____

____

____

____

35. Explain how you would help a patient to maintain or improve joint mobility.

____

____

____

____

36. Explain how walking affects joint mobility.

____

____

____

____

37. Explain how you would assist the patient to walk.

____

____

____

____

____

____

Copyright © 2019 Elsevier Canada, a division of Reed Elsevier Canada, Ltd.

Restorative and continuing care

38. Explain how the nurse would implement a plan of care to increase activity and exercise in the following specific disease conditions.
    a. Coronary heart disease: ______________________
    b. Hypertension: ______________________
    c. Chronic obstructive pulmonary disease: ______________________
    d. Diabetes mellitus: ______________________

Evaluation

Patient outcomes

Measure the effectiveness of nursing interventions by the success in meeting the patient's expected outcomes and goals of care.

39. Comparisons are made with baseline measures that include ____________, ____________, ____________, ____________, and ____________.

Patient expectations

You need to know your patient's expectations concerning activity and exercise.

REVIEW QUESTIONS

Select the appropriate answer, and cite the rationale for choosing that particular answer.

1. Which of the following is true of body mechanics?
   a. The narrower the base of support, the greater your stability.
   b. The higher the centre of gravity, the greater your stability.
   c. When friction is reduced between the object to be moved and the surface on which it is moved, less force is required to move it.
   d. Rolling, turning, or pivoting requires more work than lifting.

   Answer:__________ Rationale:__________

2. Which of the following is white, shiny, with flexible bands of fibrous tissue binding joints together and connecting various bones and cartilage?
   a. Muscles
   b. Ligaments
   c. Joints
   d. Tendons

   Answer:__________ Rationale:__________

3. Which of the following would the nurse not expect when considering the physiologic effects of exercise on the body systems?
   a. Decreased cardiac output
   b. Increased respiratory rate and depth
   c. Increased muscle tone, size, and strength
   d. Change in metabolic rate

   Answer:__________ Rationale:__________

4. Which of the following is a possible nursing diagnosis related to activity and exercise?
   a. Altered thought processes
   b. Altered oral mucous membrane
   c. Relocation stress syndrome
   d. Impaired gas exchange

   Answer:__________ Rationale:__________

CRITICAL THINKING MODEL FOR NURSING CARE PLAN FOR ACTIVITY INTOLERANCE

Imagine that you are Eric, the nurse in the Care Plan on pages 857–858 of your text. Complete the *planning* phase of the critical thinking model by writing your answers in the appropriate boxes of the model shown. Think about the following:

- In developing Mrs. Wertenberger's plan of care, what knowledge did Eric apply?
- In what way might Eric's previous experience assist in developing a plan of care for Mrs. Wertenberger?
- When developing a plan of care, what intellectual or professional standards were applied to Mrs. Wertenberger?
- What critical thinking attitudes might have been applied in developing Mrs. Wertenberger's plan?
- How will Eric accomplish his goals?

Copyright © 2019 Elsevier Canada, a division of Reed Elsevier Canada, Ltd.

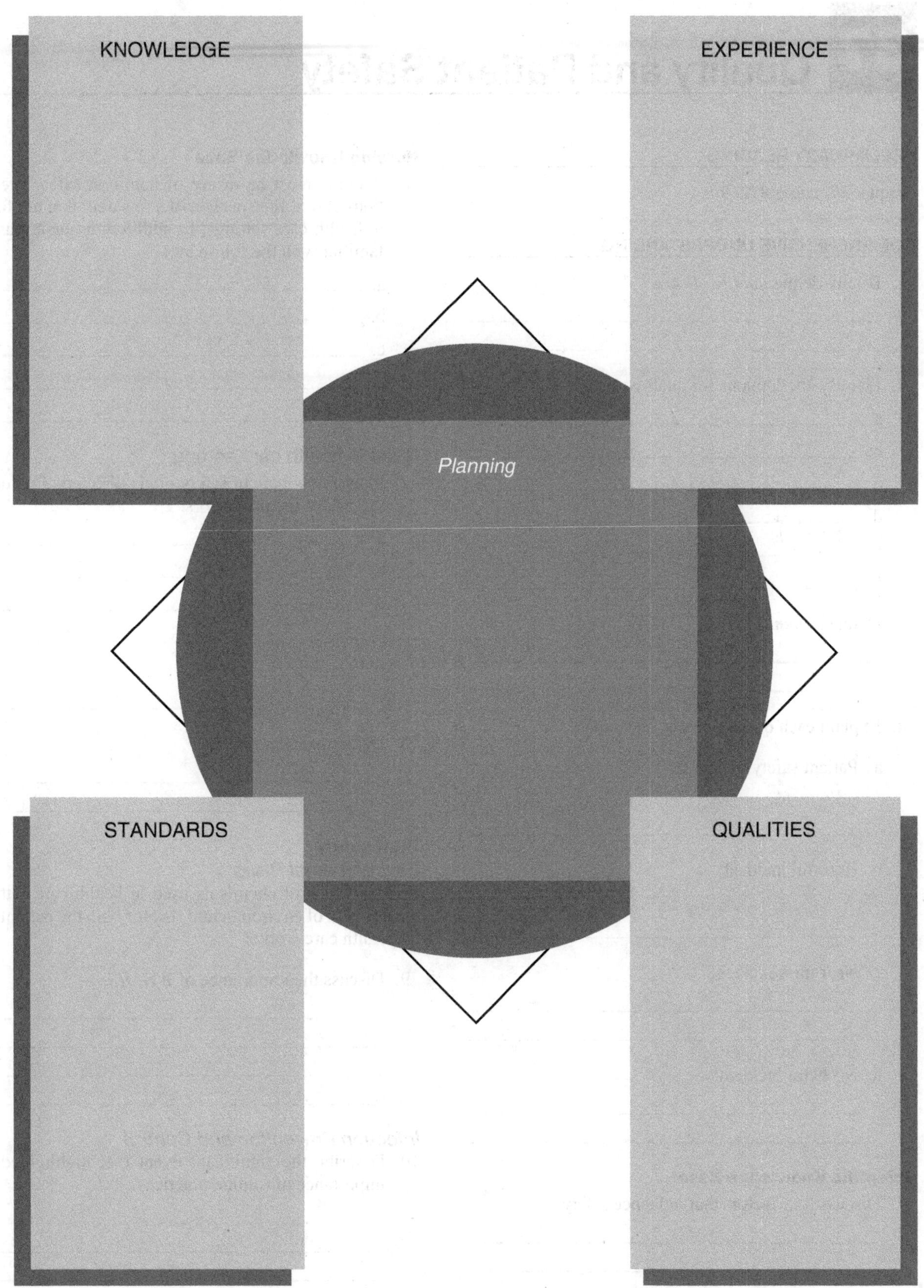

CHAPTER 36 Critical Thinking Model for Nursing Care Plan for *Activity Intolerance*
See answers on Evolve site.

Copyright © 2019 Elsevier Canada, a division of Reed Elsevier Canada, Ltd.

37 Quality and Patient Safety

PRELIMINARY READING

Chapter 37, pages 872–901

COMPREHENSIVE UNDERSTANDING

1. Briefly define *quality of care.*

2. Identify six domains for quality of care.
   a.
   b.
   c.
   d.
   e.
   f.

3. Define *patient safety.*

4. Explain each of the types of incidents.
   a. Patient safety incident:
   b. Harmful incident:
   c. Near miss incident:
   d. No-harm incident:

Scientific Knowledge Base

5. Discuss four factors that influence safety.

Nursing Knowledge Base

6. A nurse must be aware of common safety precautions and of the special risks to safety that are found in health care settings. In addition, a nurse must be familiar with the following:
   a.
   b.
   c.
   d.
   e.

Risks in health care setting

7. Identify six patient safety goals directed at reducing the risk of medical errors.
   a.
   b.
   c.
   d.
   e.
   f.

8. Define *incident report.*

Staff safety

Environmental Risks

Various forms of chemicals used in health care settings are a source of environmental risk for both the patient and the health care worker.

9. Discuss the importance of *WHMIS.*

Infection Prevention and Control

10. Describe the significant event that highlighted the importance of routine practices.

Copyright © 2019 Elsevier Canada, a division of Reed Elsevier Canada, Ltd.

Violence

11. List some factors that contribute to difficult situations.
    a. ______
    b. ______
    c. ______
    d. ______

Patient Safety

There are specific risks to a patient's safety within the health care environment and the nurse assesses for these potential problem areas.

12. Discuss some of the concerns related to patient safety.
    a. Falls:
    ______
    b. Procedure-related accidents:
    ______
    c. Equipment-related accidents:
    ______

Risks at developmental stages

13. Identify at least three threats to safety in the following developmental stages.
    a. Infant and children:
    ______
    b. Adolescents:
    ______
    c. Adulthood:
    ______
    d. Older persons:
    ______

Safety and the Nursing Process

Assessment

To conduct a thorough patient assessment, consider possible threats to the patient's safety, including the patient's immediate environment, as well as any individual risk factors.

Health history

By conducting a health history, you gather data about the patient's level of wellness to determine if any underlying conditions exist that pose threats to safety.

14. Identify the specific assessments you need to make in the patient's home.
    ______

Health care environment

15. Discuss assessment of hazards in a health care environment.
    ______
16. Explain the following health care environment risks.
    a. Risk for falls:
    ______
    b. Risk for medical errors:
    ______

Patient expectations

Patients usually do not purposefully put themselves in jeopardy. When patients are uninformed or inexperienced, threats to their safety can occur. Patients must always be consulted on ways to reduce hazards in their environment.

Nursing Process

Nursing Diagnosis

17. Identify two actual or potential nursing diagnoses for safety risks.
    a. ______
    b. ______

Planning

Goals and outcomes

18. Identify three common goals that focus on the patient's need for safety.
    a. ______
    b. ______
    c. ______

Setting priorities

19. Planning also involves understanding the patient's ______. You and the patient ______ ______ within the home and health care environment.

Copyright © 2019 Elsevier Canada, a division of Reed Elsevier Canada, Ltd.

Implementation

Nursing interventions are directed toward ensuring a patient's safety in all settings and include health promotion, developmental interventions, environmental interventions, and limiting specific risks to patient safety.

Health promotion

20. Distinguish between passive and active strategies for health promotion.

Developmental interventions

21. Identify at least four interventions for each of the following developmental age groups.

a. Infants, toddlers, preschoolers:

b. School-aged children:

c. Adolescents:

d. Adult:

e. Older persons:

Environmental interventions

Limiting Specific Risks to Patient Safety

22. List eight measures to prevent falls in the health care setting.

a.

b.

c.

d.

e.

f.

g.

h.

Restraints

23. A *restraint* is ______. The use of any type of restraint involves a psychologic adjustment for the patient and family.

24. A *physical restraint*

25. The immobility imposed by restraining a patient can lead to the following complications.

a. Physical:

b. Psychologic:

For legal purposes, know the agency's policy and procedures for the appropriate use and monitoring of physical restraints.

26. Use of restraints must meet the following objectives.

a.

b.

c.

d.

27. Distinguish between the following fall prevention devices.

a. Ambularm:

b. Bed-Check alarm:

c. Posey Bed Enclosure:

28. A *chemical restraint* is defined as

Side Rails

29. Explain the use of side rails.

Copyright © 2019 Elsevier Canada, a division of Reed Elsevier Canada, Ltd.

Electrical Hazards

30. List five guidelines for the prevention of electrical shocks.
    a. ____________________
    b. ____________________
    c. ____________________
    d. ____________________
    e. ____________________

Evaluation

Patient care

31. The nurse continually assesses the patient's and family's need for additional support services such as ____________, ____________, ____________, and ____________.

Patient expectations

32. The expected outcomes include the patient feeling ____________ and ____________ in the environment.

REVIEW QUESTIONS

Select the appropriate answer, and cite the rationale for choosing that particular answer.

1. Which of the following is *not* among the list of most common errors in hospitals?
   a. Medications
   b. Restraints
   c. Falls
   d. Early discharge

Answer:____________ Rationale:____________

2. Which developmental stage carries the highest risk of an injury from a fall?
   a. Preschool
   b. School-age
   c. Adulthood
   d. Older persons

Answer:____________ Rationale:____________

3. Mrs. Gupta falls asleep while smoking in bed and drops the burning cigarette on her blanket. When she awakens, her bed is on fire, and she quickly calls the nurse. What should the nurse immediately do upon observing the fire?
   a. Report the fire.
   b. Attempt to extinguish the fire.
   c. Assist Mrs. Gupta to a safe place.
   d. Close all windows and doors to contain the fire.

Answer:____________ Rationale:____________

4. Sixteen-year-old Simon is admitted to an adolescent unit with a diagnosis of substance abuse. The nurse examines Simon and finds that he has bloodshot eyes, slurred speech, and an unstable gait. He smells of alcohol and is unable to answer questions appropriately. What is the appropriate nursing diagnosis?
   a. Self-care deficit related to alcohol abuse
   b. Altered thought processes related to sensory overload
   c. Knowledge deficit related to alcohol abuse
   d. High risk for injury related to impaired sensory perception

Answer:____________ Rationale:____________

5. If a patient receives an electric shock, what should be your first action?
   a. Assess the patient's airway, breathing, and circulation (pulse).
   b. Assess the patient for thermal injury.
   c. Notify the physician.
   d. Notify the maintenance department.

Answer:____________ Rationale:____________

CRITICAL THINKING MODEL FOR NURSING CARE PLAN FOR RISK FOR INJURY

Imagine that you are Mr. Key, the nurse in the Care Plan on pages 881–882 of your text. Complete the *assessment* phase of the critical thinking model by writing your answers in the appropriate boxes of the model shown. Think about the following.

- In developing Ms. Cohen's plan of care, what knowledge did Mr. Key apply?
- In what way might Mr. Key's previous experience assist in this case?
- What intellectual or professional standards were applied to Ms. Cohen's case?
- What critical thinking attitudes might have been applied in this case?
- As you review your assessment, what key areas did you cover?

Copyright © 2019 Elsevier Canada, a division of Reed Elsevier Canada, Ltd.

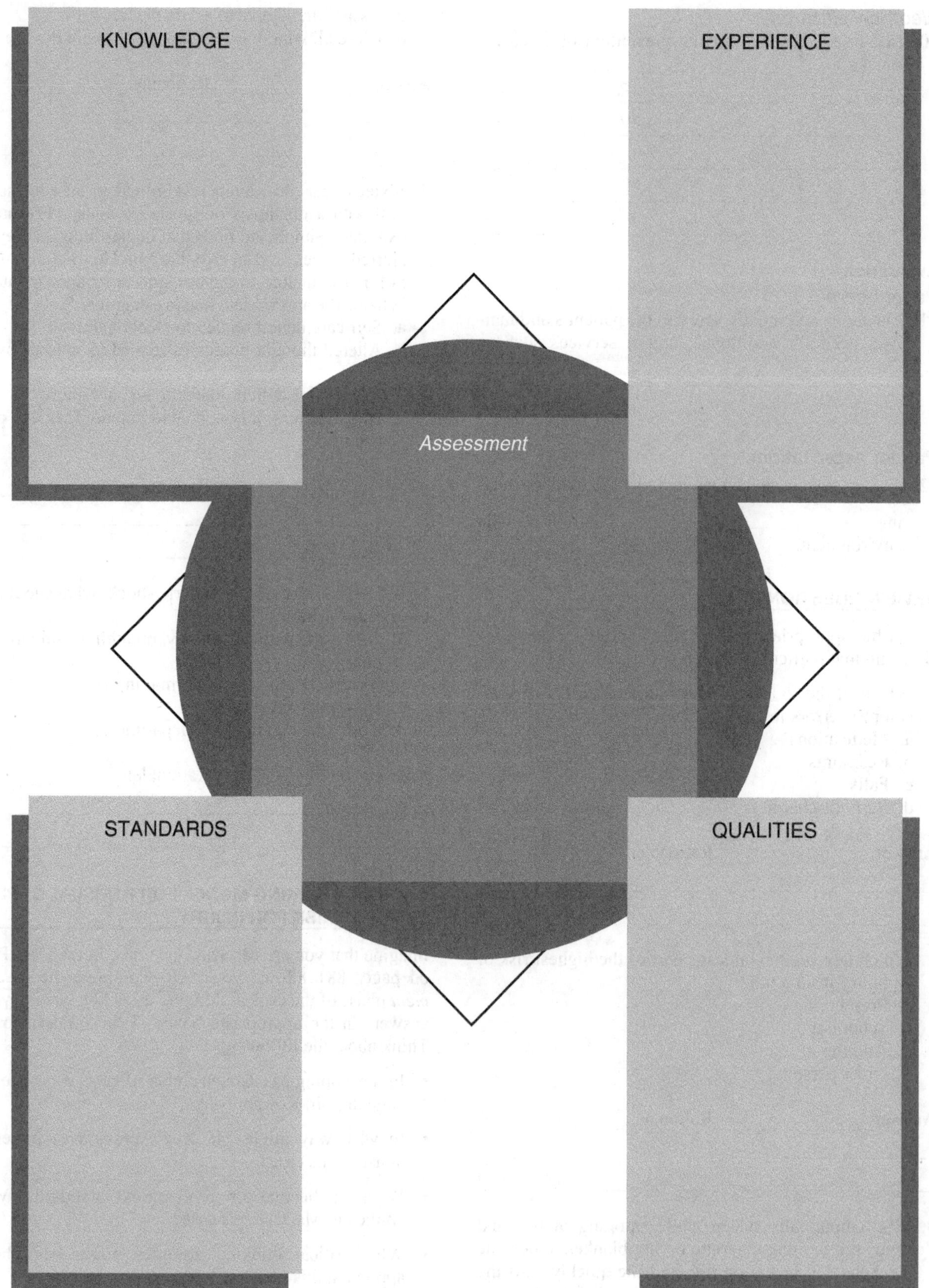

CHAPTER 37 Critical Thinking Model for Nursing Care Plan for *Risk for Injury*
See answers on Evolve site.

Copyright © 2019 Elsevier Canada, a division of Reed Elsevier Canada, Ltd.

38 Hygiene

PRELIMINARY READING

Chapter 38, pages 902–952

COMPREHENSIVE UNDERSTANDING

Personal hygiene affects an individual's comfort, safety, and physical and psychologic well-being. Individuals who are well are capable of meeting their own hygiene needs, but those who are ill or have disabilities may require various levels of assistance.

Hygiene care requires close contact with the patient; therapeutic communication skills should be used to build and promote a caring therapeutic relationship and to assist you in providing the patient with teaching regarding hygiene care.

Scientific Knowledge Base

Proper hygiene care requires an understanding of the anatomy and physiology of the integument, oral cavity, eyes, ears, nose, hands, feet, and nails. Good hygiene techniques assist in promoting the normal structure and function of body tissues.

The skin

1. Identify the functions of the skin.

 ____

 ____

 ____

2. The skin has three primary layers, as follows:

 a. ______________________

 b. ______________________

 c. ______________________

3. Bacteria commonly reside on the outer layer of skin (the *epidermis*). These resident bacteria are normal flora; they do not __________ but instead __________ of disease-causing microorganisms.

The skin can provide crucial information regarding a patient's health status and provide important information regarding the functioning of other systems and organs.

The feet, hands, and nails

The feet, hands, and nails often require special attention to prevent infection.

4. Define the following terms.

 a. *Cuticle*:

 ____

 ____

 b. *Lunula*:

 ____

 ____

 c. *Nail bed*:

 ____

 ____

The oral cavity

The oral cavity extends from the lips to the anterior pillars of the tonsils. It is the structure for taste, mastication, and speech articulation.

5. The *buccal mucosa* (oral mucosa) are normally __________ and __________.

6. The mouth also contains three pairs of salivary glands that start the digestive process by releasing enzymes that perform the following:

 a. ______________________

 b. ______________________

 c. ______________________

Salivary secretion can be decreased by medications and disease processes.

7. Teeth are organs of chewing, or __________, and are designed to __________.

8. Regular oral hygiene is necessary to maintain the integrity of tooth surfaces and to prevent __________ __________.

The hair

9. Identify the factors that can affect the hair's characteristics.

 ____

 ____

The eyes, ears, and nose

Cleansing of the sensitive sensory tissues should be done in a way to prevent injury and patient discomfort.

Nursing Knowledge Base

No two individuals perform hygiene in the same manner, and it is important to individualize care from knowledge about the patient's unique hygiene practices and preferences.

Copyright © 2019 Elsevier Canada, a division of Reed Elsevier Canada, Ltd.

10. Briefly explain each of the following factors influencing hygiene habits.

    a. Social practices:

    b. Personal preferences:

    c. Body image:

    d. Socioeconomic status:

    e. Health beliefs and motivation:

    f. Cultural variables:

    g. Physical condition:

Critical Thinking

Hygiene care is so important for patients to feel comfortable, refreshed, and renewed; you should avoid making hygiene care a simple routine. Instead, integrate knowledge from nursing and other disciplines, previous experiences, and information gathered from patients.

The Nursing Process

Assessment

Important considerations include assessment of the patient's ability to perform self-care, usual hygiene practices and preferences, with special attention to balance, coordination, strength, range of motion, and activity tolerance.

Physical examination

Nurses utilize the skills of inspection and palpation; look for alterations in the integrity and function of tissues.

The Skin

11. When inspecting the skin, the nurse thoroughly examines the following:

    a.

    b.

    c.

    d.

    e.

    f.

12. Common skin problems can affect how hygiene is administered. Describe the hygiene provided for the following:

    a. Dry skin:

    b. Acne:

    c. Skin rashes:

    d. Contact dermatitis:

    e. Psoriasis:

    f. Abrasion:

13. Briefly explain the six conditions that place patients at risk for impaired skin integrity.

    a. Immobilization:

    b. Reduced sensation:

Copyright © 2019 Elsevier Canada, a division of Reed Elsevier Canada, Ltd.

c. Nutrition and hydration alterations:

d. Secretions and excretions on the skin:

e. Vascular insufficiency:

f. External devices:

The Feet and Nails

Assessment of the feet involves a thorough examination of all skin surfaces, including the soles of the feet and the areas between the toes.

14. Inspection of the feet for lesions includes noting areas of:
    a.
    b.
    c.

15. Define *neuropathy.*

16. Describe a nursing assessment for neuropathy.

17. Identify the characteristics of the following foot and nail problems.
    a. Calluses:
    b. Keratosis (corn):
    c. Plantar warts:
    d. Athlete's foot (tinea pedis):
    e. Ingrown nails:
    f. Ram's horn nails:
    g. Paronychia:
    h. Foot odour:

The Oral Cavity

18. The nurse inspects all areas of the oral cavity for the following:
    a.
    b.
    c.
    d.

19. Define the following terms.
    a. *Halitosis*:
    b. *Stomatitis*:

The Hair

20. Describe the characteristics of the following hair and scalp conditions.
    a. Dandruff:
    b. Ticks:
    c. Pediculosis capitis (head lice):
    d. Pediculosis corporis (body lice):

Copyright © 2019 Elsevier Canada, a division of Reed Elsevier Canada, Ltd.

e. Pediculosis pubis (crab lice):

f. Alopecia (hair loss):

The Eyes, Ears, and Nose

21. Identify the normal assessment findings for the following:

a. Eyes:

b. Ears:

c. Nose:

Developmental changes

The Skin

22. For each developmental stage, briefly describe normal conditions that create a high risk for impaired skin integrity.

a. Neonate:

b. Toddler:

c. Adolescent:

d. Older person:

The Feet and Nails

23. Identify the common foot problems of the older persons.

The Oral Cavity

24. Identify factors associated with aging that can result in poor oral care.

The Eyes, Ears, and Nose

As patients age, they are also at risk for changes in visual clarity and visual field losses.

25. Older persons experience the following auditory changes as the result of aging.

a. ______

b. ______

c. ______

Changes in smell seem to be more common in older persons. These changes may also affect taste and appetite.

Self-care ability

26. Identify factors that are assessed to determine a patient's ability to perform routine hygiene.

When a patient has self-care limitations, part of the assessment is to determine whether family or friends are available to assist.

Hygiene practices

Asking the patient to assist or teach how to perform preferred grooming practices gives the patient a greater sense of independence and helps you to avoid causing the patient discomfort or injury.

Cultural factors

27. Explain how culture affects a patient's hygiene needs.

Copyright © 2019 Elsevier Canada, a division of Reed Elsevier Canada, Ltd.

Patients at risk for hygiene problems

28. Provide examples of patients at risk for the following problems.

   a. Oral problems:

   ______

   b. Skin problems:

   ______

   c. Foot problems:

   ______

   d. Eye care problems:

   ______

Special considerations in hygiene assessment

29. Explain how footwear may predispose a patient to foot and nail problems.

   ______

Nursing Diagnosis

30. List four possible nursing diagnoses that apply to patients in need of hygiene care.

   a. ______
   b. ______
   c. ______
   d. ______

Planning

During planning, you synthesize information from multiple resources.

Goals and outcomes

31. When providing for patient hygiene, you care for a variety of patients with different self-care abilities and needs. List three possible outcomes.

   a. ______
   b. ______
   c. ______

Setting priorities

The patient's condition influences the plan for delivering hygiene.

Implementation

32. The use of ______ helps to ______ and promote ______ while you perform each hygiene measure.

Health promotion

33. List four guidelines for educating patients about hygiene care.

   a. ______
   b. ______
   c. ______
   d. ______

Acute and restorative care

34. Compare and contrast the four types of scheduled care in acute and long-term settings.

   a. ______
   b. ______
   c. ______
   d. ______

Bathing and skin care

The extent of patients' baths and the methods used for bathing depend on their physical abilities, health problems, and the degree of hygiene required.

35. A complete bed bath is ______.

36. A partial bed bath involves ______.

37. Identify guidelines the nurse should follow when assisting or providing a patient with any type of bath.

   ______

Bag Baths

38. Describe what a bag bath is, and why it may be preferred over wash basins.

   ______

Copyright © 2019 Elsevier Canada, a division of Reed Elsevier Canada, Ltd.

Perineal Care

39. Define *perineal care*, and identify the patients at risk for skin breakdown in the perineal area.

Back Rub

40. A back rub promotes the following:
    a.
    b.
    c.
    d.
    e.
    f.
    g.

Foot and Nail Care

41. List at least eight guidelines to include when advising patients with peripheral neuropathy or vascular insufficiency about foot care.
    a.
    b.
    c.
    d.
    e.
    f.
    g.
    h.

Oral hygiene

42. Oral hygiene helps to maintain ______________.
43. Briefly explain the following interventions in relation to oral hygiene.
    a. Diet:

    b. Brushing and flossing:

    c. Oral care for patients with special needs:

    d. Denture care:

Hair and scalp care

44. Briefly describe the rationales for the following:
    a. Brushing and combing:

    b. Shampooing:

    c. Shaving:

    d. Moustache and beard care:

Care of the eyes, ears, and nose

Care focuses on preventing infection and maintaining normal sensory function.

Basic Eye Care

45. Describe basic eye care for a patient.

Eyeglasses

46. Describe the correct procedure for cleaning eyeglasses.

Copyright © 2019 Elsevier Canada, a division of Reed Elsevier Canada, Ltd.

Contact Lenses

47. Briefly describe proper contact lens care technique.

Artificial Eyes

48. Describe each of the following techniques necessary in caring for an artificial eye.
    a. Removal:
    b. Cleansing:
    c. Reinsertion:
    d. Storage:

Ear Care

49. Describe the procedure for removing cerumen from the ear.

Hearing Aid Care

50. Describe the following types of hearing aids.
    a. In-the-canal:
    b. In-the-ear:
    c. Behind-the-ear:

Nasal Care

51. Describe three interventions used to remove secretions from the nose.
    a.
    b.
    c.

Patient's room environment

Maintaining Comfort

52. Identify four factors the nurse can control to create a more comfortable environment.
    a.
    b.
    c.
    d.

Room Equipment

53. A typical hospital room contains the following basic pieces of furniture.
    a.
    b.
    c.
    d.

Beds

54. A patient's bed must be frequently inspected to ensure that the linens are ______, ______, and ______.
55. Identify the factors a nurse considers when making a patient's bed.

Evaluation

Patient care

Evaluation of hygiene measures occurs before, during, and after each particular skill.

The standards for evaluation are the expected outcomes established in the planning stage of the patient's care.

Patient expectations

The patient's expectations are important guidelines in determining patient satisfaction.

Copyright © 2019 Elsevier Canada, a division of Reed Elsevier Canada, Ltd.

REVIEW QUESTIONS

Select the appropriate answer, and cite the rationale for choosing that particular answer.

1. Mr. Ng is a 19-year-old patient in the rehabilitation unit. He is completely paralyzed below the neck. What is the most appropriate bath for Mr. Ng?
   a. Partial bed bath
   b. Complete bed bath
   c. Sitz bath
   d. Tepid bath

Answer: ______________ Rationale: ______________

____

____

2. Which of the following will *not* help maintain skin integrity in the older person?
   a. Environmental air that is cold and dry
   b. Use of warm water and mild cleansing agents for bathing
   c. Bathing every other day
   d. Drinking 8 to 10 glasses of water a day

Answer: ______________ Rationale: ______________

____

____

3. When preparing to give complete morning care to a patient, what would the nurse do first?
   a. Gather the necessary equipment and supplies.
   b. Remove the patient's gown or pyjamas while maintaining privacy.
   c. Assess the patient's preferences for bathing practices.
   d. Lower the side rails, and assist the patient to assume a comfortable position.

Answer: ______________ Rationale: ______________

____

____

4. Mrs. Veech has diabetes. Which intervention should be included in her teaching plan regarding foot care?
   a. Use a pumice stone to smooth corns and calluses.
   b. File toenails straight across and square.
   c. Apply powder to dry areas along the feet and between the toes.
   d. Wear elastic stockings to improve circulation.

Answer: ______________ Rationale: ______________

____

____

5. Assessment of the hair and scalp reveals that a patient has pediculosis capitis. What is an appropriate intervention?
   a. Shave hair off the affected area.
   b. Place oil on the hair and scalp until all of the lice are dead.
   c. Use a medicated shampoo, and repeat 7 to 10 days later.
   d. Shampoo with regular shampoo, and dry with the hair dryer set at the hottest setting.

Answer: ______________ Rationale: ______________

____

____

CRITICAL THINKING MODEL FOR NURSING CARE PLAN FOR INEFFECTIVE TISSUE PERFUSION, IMPROPER FOOT CARE, AND HYGIENE

Imagine that you are the nurse in the Care Plan on page 916 of your text. Complete the *planning* phase of the critical thinking model by writing your answers in the appropriate boxes of the model shown. Think about the following.

- In developing Mr. James's plan of care, what knowledge did you apply?
- In what way might your previous experience assist in developing a plan of care for Mr. James?
- When developing a plan of care, what intellectual and professional standards were applied?
- What critical thinking attitudes might have been applied in developing Mr. James's plan of care?
- How will you accomplish the goals?

Copyright © 2019 Elsevier Canada, a division of Reed Elsevier Canada, Ltd.

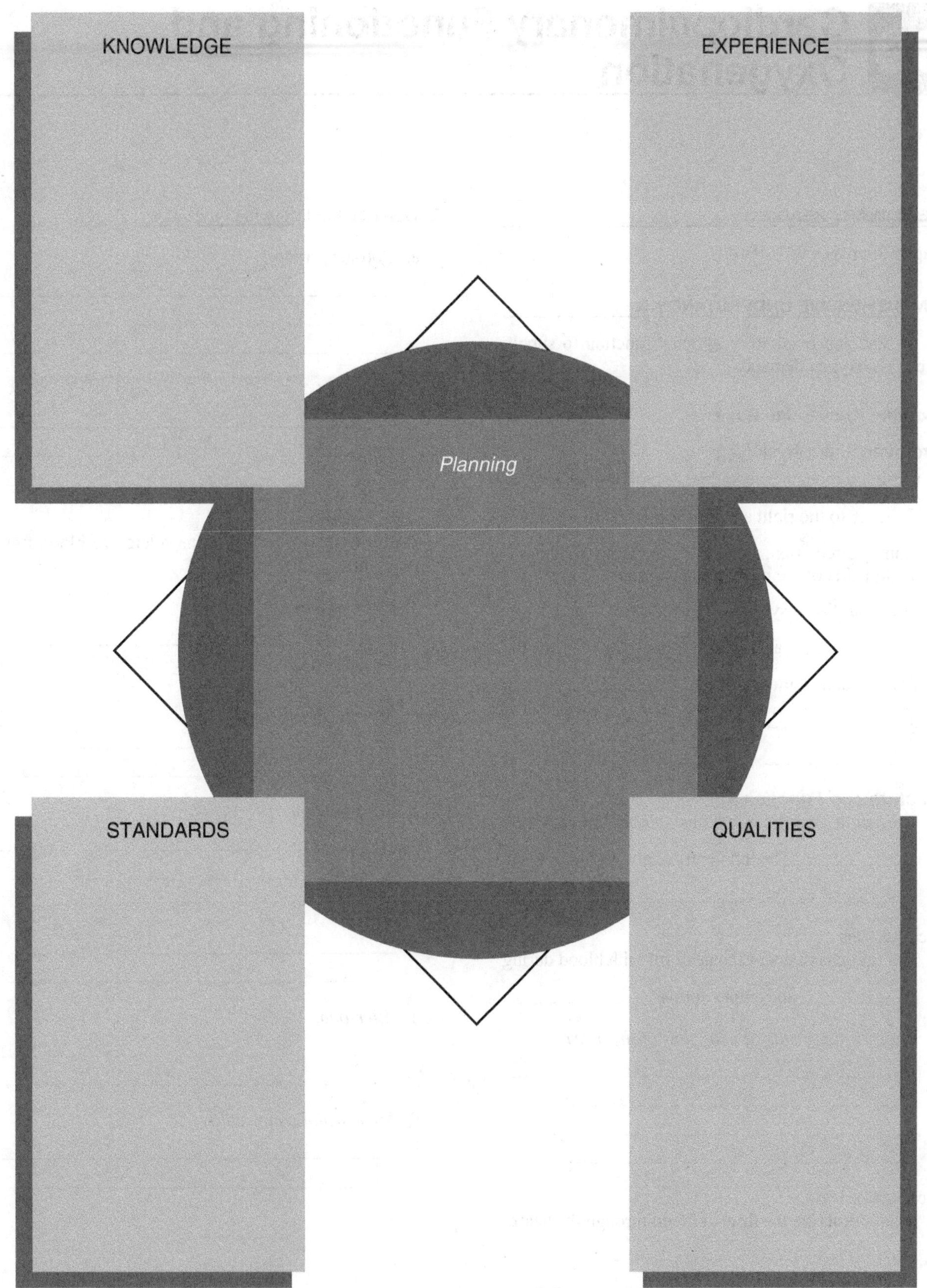

CHAPTER 38 Critical Thinking Model for Nursing Care Plan for *Ineffective Tissue Perfusion, Improper Foot Care, and Hygiene*
See answers on Evolve site.

Copyright © 2019 Elsevier Canada, a division of Reed Elsevier Canada, Ltd.

39 Cardiopulmonary Functioning and Oxygenation

PRELIMINARY READING

Chapter 39, pages 953–1014

COMPREHENSIVE UNDERSTANDING

The cardiac and respiratory systems function to supply the body's oxygen demands.

Scientific Knowledge Base

Cardiovascular physiology

1. Cardiopulmonary physiology involves delivery of _______ to the right side of the heart and to the pulmonary circulation, and _________ from the lungs to the left side of the heart and the tissues.
2. The cardiac system delivers ___________, ___________, and other ___________ to the tissues, and removes the ___________ through the ___________, ___________, and ___________ ___________.

Structure and Function

3. The right ventricle pumps blood through the ___________. The left ventricle pumps blood to the ___________.

Myocardial Pump

4. The four chambers of the heart fill with blood during ___________ and empty during ___________.
5. Describe the *Frank-Starling law of the heart.*

Myocardial Blood Flow

6. Briefly describe the flow of blood through the heart.
7. Describe the following types of circulation.
   a. Coronary artery:
   b. Systemic:

Blood Flow Regulation

8. Describe the following terms related to blood flow regulation.
   a. *Cardiac output:*
   b. *Cardiac index:*
   c. *Stroke volume:*
   d. *Preload:*
   e. *Afterload:*
   f. *Myocardial contractility:*

Copyright © 2019 Elsevier Canada, a division of Reed Elsevier Canada, Ltd.

Conduction System

The rhythmic relaxation and contraction of the atria and ventricles depend on continuous, organized transmission of electrical impulses.

9. Describe how the following affect the conduction system of the heart.

   a. Sympathetic nerve fibres:

   ____

   ____

   ____

   ____

   b. Parasympathetic nerve fibres:

   ____

   ____

   ____

   ____

10. Diagram and label the electrical conduction system of the heart in the box provided.

Copyright © 2019 Elsevier Canada, a division of Reed Elsevier Canada, Ltd.

11. Diagram and label the components of the electrocardiogram (ECG) waveform for normal sinus rhythm in the box provided.

Respiratory physiology

12. The three steps in the process of oxygenation are __________, __________, and __________.

Structure and Function

13. The __________, __________, __________, and __________ are essential for ventilation, perfusion, and exchange of respiratory gases.

14. Define *ventilation.*

____
____
____

Work of Breathing

Breathing is the effort required for expanding and contracting the lungs.

15. __________ is an __________ process, stimulated by chemical receptors in the aorta. __________ is a __________ process that depends on the elastic-recoil properties of the lungs, requiring little or no muscle work.

16. Define the following terms related to the work of breathing.

a. *Surfactant*:

____
____
____

b. *Accessory muscles*:

____
____
____

c. *Compliance*:

____
____
____

Copyright © 2019 Elsevier Canada, a division of Reed Elsevier Canada, Ltd.

d. *Airway resistance*: ______

Lung Volumes and Capacities

17. Spirometry is used to ______.

18. Variations in lung volumes may be associated with health states such as ______, ______, ______, or ______ and ______ conditions of the lungs.

19. The amount of ______, ______, and ______ can affect pressures and volumes within the lungs.

Pulmonary Circulation

20. Briefly describe *the pulmonary circulation.*

21. Identify the normal distribution of pressures within the pulmonary circulation.

Respiratory Gas Exchange

22. Respiratory gases are exchanged in the ______ and the ______ of the body tissues.

23. Define *diffusion.*

24. How can the rate of diffusion be affected?

Oxygen Transport

25. List four factors required for oxygen transport and delivery.
    a. ______
    b. ______
    c. ______
    d. ______

Carbon Dioxide Transport

26. Describe the breakdown of carbon dioxide as it is diffused into the red blood cells.

Regulation of Respiration

27. Explain the two regulators that control the process of respiration.
    a. Neural:
    b. Chemical:

Factors affecting oxygenation

28. List the four factors that influence oxygenation.
    a. ______
    b. ______
    c. ______
    d. ______

Physiologic Factors

29. Explain the following factors that affect the body's ability to meet oxygen demands. Give examples of each.
    a. Decreased oxygen-carrying capacity:
    b. Decreased inspired oxygen concentration:
    c. Hypovolemia:

Copyright © 2019 Elsevier Canada, a division of Reed Elsevier Canada, Ltd.

d. Increased metabolic rate:

___

___

___

Conditions Affecting Chest Wall Movement

30. Explain how the following conditions affect chest wall movement.

a. Pregnancy:

___

b. Obesity:

___

c. Musculoskeletal abnormalities:

___

d. Trauma:

___

e. Neuromuscular diseases:

___

f. Central nervous system alterations:

___

g. Influences of chronic disease:

___

Alterations in cardiac functioning

31. Illnesses and conditions that affect ___, ___, ___, ___, and ___ cause alterations in cardiac functioning.

Disturbances in Conduction

32. Define *dysrhythmias*.

___

33. Briefly describe the following dysrhythmias.

a. *Sinus tachycardia*:

___

b. *Sinus bradycardia*:

___

c. *Atrial fibrillation*:

___

d. *Ventricular tachycardia*:

___

e. *Ventricular fibrillation*:

___

f. *Asystole*:

___

Altered Cardiac Output

34. Failure of the myocardium to eject sufficient volume to the systemic and pulmonary circulations can result in left-sided and right-sided heart failure. Complete the following grid.

Type of Heart Failure	Clinical Findings
Left-sided	
Right-sided	

Copyright © 2019 Elsevier Canada, a division of Reed Elsevier Canada, Ltd.

Impaired Valvular Function

35. Define each of the following terms.

    a. *Valvular heart disease*:

    b. *Stenosis*:

    c. *Regurgitation*:

    d. *Myocardial ischemia*:

    e. *Angina pectoris*:

    f. *Myocardial infarction*:

36. Describe the chest pain associated with myocardial infarction.

Acute Coronary Syndrome

37. Briefly explain *acute coronary syndrome.*

Alterations in respiratory functioning

38. The three primary alterations in respiratory function are ________, ________, and ________.

39. Complete the following grid to identify the causes, signs, and symptoms of alterations in respiratory functioning.

Alterations	Causes	Signs and Symptoms
Hyperventilation		
Hypoventilation		
Hypoxia		

40. Define the following terms.

    a. *Atelectasis*:

    b. *Cyanosis*:

Nursing Knowledge Base

Developmental factors

41. Identify at least one physiologic factor influencing tissue oxygenation for each developmental level listed.

    a. Infants and toddlers:

    b. School-age children and adolescents:

Copyright © 2019 Elsevier Canada, a division of Reed Elsevier Canada, Ltd.

c. Young and middle-aged adults:

d. Older persons:

Lifestyle risk factors

42. Briefly describe how the following lifestyle factors influence respiratory function.

a. Poor nutrition:

b. Inadequate exercise:

c. Smoking:

d. Substance abuse:

e. Stress:

Environmental factors

43. List four occupational pollutants.

a.

b.

c.

d.

Nursing Process

Assessment

44. Briefly describe health history for the following:

a. Cardiac function:

b. Respiratory function:

45. Define the following terms.

a. *Fatigue*:

b. *Dyspnea*:

c. *Orthopnea*:

d. *Cough*:

e. *Productive cough*:

f. *Hemoptysis*:

g. *Wheezing*:

Copyright © 2019 Elsevier Canada, a division of Reed Elsevier Canada, Ltd.

46. Briefly explain why special considerations are necessary for older persons during the physical examination.

47. Briefly explain the following techniques used during the physical examination to assess tissue oxygenation.

a. Inspection:

b. Palpation:

c. Percussion:

d. Auscultation:

Diagnostic tests

48. Describe the following tests that determine myocardial contraction and blood flow.

a. Echocardiography:

b. Scintigraphy:

c. Cardiac catheterization and angiography:

49. Describe the following diagnostic tests used to determine the adequacy of the cardiac conduction system.

a. Electrocardiogram:

b. Holter monitor:

c. ECG exercise stress test:

d. Thallium stress test:

50. Describe the following tests used to measure the adequacy of ventilation and oxygenation.

a. Pulse oximetry:

b. Arterial blood gases:

c. Pulmonary function tests:

d. Chest X-ray examination:

e. Computed tomography scan:

f. Ventilation/perfusion (nuclear medicine) lung scan:

51. Describe the following tests used to determine abnormal cells or infection in the respiratory tract.

a. Sputum tests:

b. Bronchoscopy:

c. Thoracentesis:

Copyright © 2019 Elsevier Canada, a division of Reed Elsevier Canada, Ltd.

d. Nasopharyngeal aspirate or swab: ______

Nursing Diagnosis

Patients with an altered level of oxygenation can have nursing diagnoses that are primarily from a cardiovascular or pulmonary origin.

Planning

Goals and outcomes

52. List four goals appropriate for a patient with actual or potential oxygenation needs.

a. ______
b. ______
c. ______
d. ______

Implementation

Health promotion

Vaccinations

53. Describe the purpose of the influenza and pneumococcal vaccines, and explain for whom the vaccines are recommended.

______

Healthy Lifestyle Behaviour

54. Identify some healthy lifestyle behaviours that decrease the risk of cardiopulmonary disease.

______

Acute care

55. Nursing interventions for the patient with acute pulmonary illnesses are directed toward ______, ______, and ______.

Dyspnea Management

56. List four treatment modalities appropriate for a patient with dyspnea.

a. ______
b. ______
c. ______
d. ______

Airway Maintenance

The airway is patent when the trachea, bronchi, and large airways are free from obstructions.

Mobilization of Pulmonary Secretions

57. Nursing interventions that promote mobilization of pulmonary secretions include the following factors. Briefly explain each one.

a. *Humidification*: ______

b. *Nebulization*: ______

c. *Chest physiotherapy (CPT)*: ______

58. Briefly describe the three activities involved in CPT.

a. Chest percussion: ______

b. Vibration: ______

c. Postural drainage: ______

Suctioning Techniques

Suctioning is necessary when a patient is unable to clear respiratory tract secretions with coughing.

59. Briefly explain the following types of suctioning techniques.

a. Oropharyngeal and nasopharyngeal: ______

Copyright © 2019 Elsevier Canada, a division of Reed Elsevier Canada, Ltd.

b. Orotracheal and nasotracheal:

c. Tracheal:

Maintenance and Promotion of Lung Expansion

60. Nursing interventions that maintain or promote lung expansion include the following noninvasive techniques. Briefly explain each.

a. Positioning:

b. Incentive spirometry:

Chest Tubes

61. Identify the three reasons for inserting chest tubes.

a.

b.

c.

62. Define the following terms.

a. *Pneumothorax*:

b. *Hemothorax*:

63. Discuss the two types of drainage devices used with chest tubes.

a.

b.

Special Considerations

64. Identify five special considerations the nurse needs to address when dealing with chest tubes.

a.

b.

c.

d.

e.

Maintenance and Promotion of Oxygenation

Promotion of lung expansion, mobilization of secretions, and maintenance of a patent airway assist the patient in meeting oxygenation needs.

65. Identify the goal of oxygen therapy.

Safety Precautions

66. List five safety measures to institute when a patient receives oxygen.

a.

b.

c.

d.

e.

Methods of Oxygen Delivery

67. Describe the following methods of oxygen delivery, and identify the usual flow rates.

a. Nasal cannula:

b. Face mask:

c. Partial-rebreathing mask and the non-rebreathing mask:

d. Venturi mask:

Copyright © 2019 Elsevier Canada, a division of Reed Elsevier Canada, Ltd.

Home Oxygen Therapy

68. Identify the indications for a patient to receive home oxygen therapy.

______

69. Identify the teaching required by the patient for use of home oxygen therapy.

______

Restoration of Cardiopulmonary Functioning

If a patient's hypoxia is severe and prolonged, cardiac arrest may result. Permanent heart, brain, and other tissue damage occur within 4 to 6 minutes.

Cardiopulmonary Resuscitation (CPR)

70. List the sequence of steps for CPR.

a. ______

b. ______

c. ______

Restorative and continuing care

71. Cardiopulmonary rehabilitation is ______.

Hydration

Maintenance of adequate systemic hydration keeps mucociliary clearance normal.

Coughing Techniques

72. Coughing is effective for maintaining a patent airway. List four coughing techniques.

a. ______

b. ______

c. ______

d. ______

Respiratory Muscle Training

Respiratory muscle training improves muscle strength and endurance, resulting in improved activity tolerance.

Breathing Exercises

73. Briefly explain the following breathing exercises used to improve ventilation and oxygenation.

a. *Pursed-lip breathing*:

______

b. *Diaphragmatic breathing*:

______

Evaluation

Patient care

The nurse evaluates the actual care provided to the patient by the health care team based on the expected outcomes.

The patient is the only person who can evaluate his or her degree of breathlessness.

74. The evaluation of ______ and ______ are done by comparing the patient's ______ with the goals and ______ of the nursing care plan.

Patient expectations

Evaluate the care from the patient's perspective.

Working closely with the patient will enable the nurse to redefine those patient expectations that can be realistically met within the limitations of the patient's condition and treatment.

REVIEW QUESTIONS

Select the appropriate answer, and cite the rationale for choosing that particular answer.

1. Which function includes ventilation, perfusion, and the exchange of gases?
   a. Respiration
   b. Circulation
   c. Aerobic metabolism
   d. Anaerobic metabolism

Answer: ______ Rationale: ______

2. Which of the following best describes *afterload*?
   a. The amount of blood ejected from the left ventricle each minute
   b. The amount of blood ejected from the left ventricle with each contraction
   c. The resistance to left ventricle ejection
   d. The amount of blood in the left ventricle

Answer: ______ Rationale: ______

Copyright © 2019 Elsevier Canada, a division of Reed Elsevier Canada, Ltd.

3. What does the movement of gases into and out of the lungs depend upon?
   a. 50% oxygen content in the atmospheric air
   b. Pressure gradient between the atmosphere and the alveoli
   c. Use of accessory muscles of respiration during expiration
   d. Amount of carbon dioxide dissolved in the fluid of the alveoli

Answer:_______________ Rationale:_______________

____

____

4. A nurse who is analyzing the patient's ECG sees that it shows a regular rhythm with a rate of 140 to 160 beats per minute and that the P-wave and QRS complex are normal. What is this rhythm called?
   a. Sinus tachycardia
   b. Sinus dysrhythmia
   c. Supraventricular tachycardia
   d. Premature ventricular contractions

Answer:_______________ Rationale:_______________

____

____

5. Mr. Isaac comes to the emergency department complaining of difficulty breathing. Which objective assessment would relate to his dyspnea?
   a. Statements about a sense of impending doom
   b. Complaints of shortness of breath
   c. Feelings of heaviness in the chest
   d. Use of accessory muscles of respiration

Answer:_______________ Rationale:_______________

____

____

6. What is used when performing chest physiotherapy to mobilize pulmonary secretions?
   a. Hydration
   b. Percussion
   c. Nebulization
   d. Humidification

Answer:_______________ Rationale:_______________

____

____

CRITICAL THINKING MODEL FOR NURSING CARE PLAN FOR INEFFECTIVE AIRWAY CLEARANCE/ RETAINED SECRETIONS

Imagine that you are the student nurse in the Care Plan on page 976 of your text. Complete the assessment phase of the critical thinking model by writing your answers in the appropriate boxes of the model shown. Think about the following:

- What knowledge base was applied to Mr. Edwards?
- In what way might your previous experience apply in this case?
- What intellectual or professional standards were applied to Mr. Edwards?
- What critical thinking attitudes did you use in assessing Mr. Edwards?
- As you review your assessment, what key areas did you cover?

Copyright © 2019 Elsevier Canada, a division of Reed Elsevier Canada, Ltd.

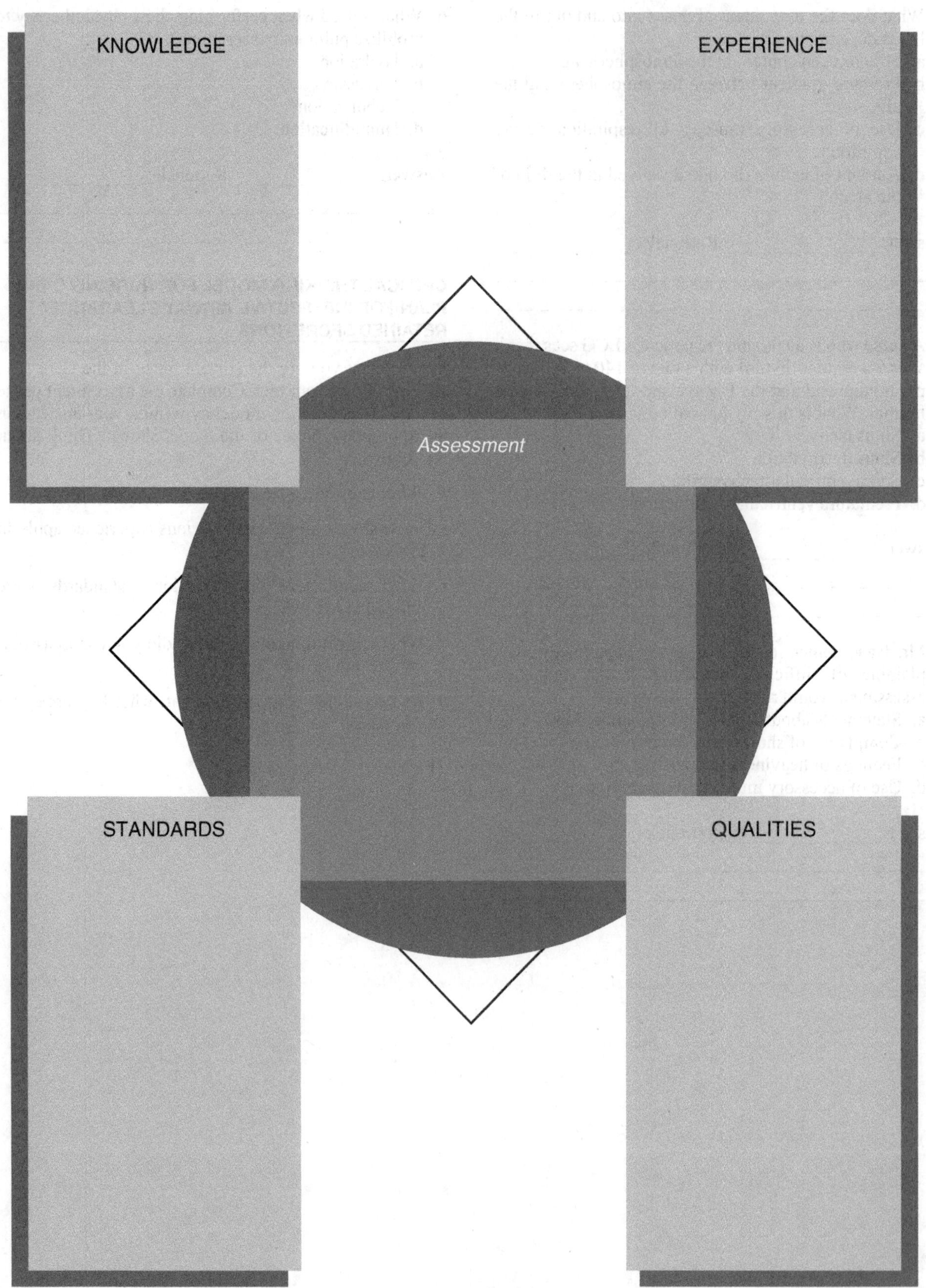

CHAPTER 39 Critical Thinking Model for Nursing Care Plan for *Ineffective Airway Clearance/Retained Secretions*
See answers on Evolve site.

Copyright © 2019 Elsevier Canada, a division of Reed Elsevier Canada, Ltd.

40 Fluid, Electrolyte, and Acid–Base Balances

PRELIMINARY READING

Chapter 40, pages 1015–1071

COMPREHENSIVE UNDERSTANDING

Fluid, electrolyte, and acid–base balances within the body are essential for normal body function.

Scientific Knowledge Base

1. ______________ is the largest single component of the body, 60% of the average adult's weight.

Distribution of body fluids

2. Body fluids are distributed in two distinct compartments. Briefly explain each one.

   a. Extracellular fluid (ECF):

   b. Intracellular fluid (ICF):

3. ECFs are divided into three smaller compartments. Explain each.

   a. Interstitial fluid:

   b. Intravascular fluid:

   c. Transcellular fluid:

Composition of body fluids

4. Define *electrolytes*.

5. Define the following terms related to the composition of body fluids.

   a. *Cations*:

   b. *Anions*:

   c. *mmol/L*:

   d. *Solute*:

   e. *Solvent*:

   f. *Minerals*:

Movement of body fluids

Fluids and electrolytes constantly shift between compartments to facilitate body processes.

6. List and briefly describe the four factors responsible for the movement of body fluids.

   a.

   b.

   c.

   d.

Copyright © 2019 Elsevier Canada, a division of Reed Elsevier Canada, Ltd.

Osmosis

7. Define the following terms related to osmosis.
   a. *Osmotic pressure*: ________________
   b. *Colloid osmotic pressure or oncotic pressure*: ________________
8. Define *hydrostatic pressure*. ________________

Carrier-Mediated Transport

9. *Carrier-mediated transport* moves molecules across the plasma membrane. Give two examples of carrier-mediated transport.
   a. ________________
   b. ________________

Regulation of body fluids

10. Body fluids are regulated by ________, ________, and ________. This balance is termed ________.

Fluid Output Regulation

11. Fluid output occurs through four organs. List and explain each one.
    a. ________________
    b. ________________
    c. ________________
    d. ________________

Fluid Intake Regulation

12. Briefly describe the physiologic stimuli triggering the thirst mechanism. ________________

Hormonal Regulation of Fluid

13. For each hormone in the grid provided, identify the stimuli for its release and its influence on fluid and electrolyte balance.

Hormone	Stimuli	Action
Antidiuretic hormone		
Aldosterone		

Regulation of electrolytes

For normal cell function and human well-being, the body maintains a normal balance of electrolytes in the ECF and ICF despite changes in intake and loss.

14. The major cations within the body fluids include ________, ________, ________, and ________.
15. The major anions are ________, ________, and ________.
16. Give the normal values, function, and regulatory mechanisms for the major body electrolytes in the following grid.

Electrolyte	Normal Value	Function	Regulatory Mechanism
Sodium			
Potassium			
Calcium			
Magnesium			

Copyright © 2019 Elsevier Canada, a division of Reed Elsevier Canada, Ltd.

Electrolyte	Normal Value	Function	Regulatory Mechanism
Chloride			
Bicarbonate			
Phosphate			

Regulation of acid–base balance

Acid–base balance exists when the rate at which the body produces and gains acids or bases, through cellular metabolism and gastrointestinal (GI) absorption, equals the rate at which acids or bases are excreted.

17. A ____________ is a substance or a group of substances, such as ____________, ____________, and ____________ that can absorb or release hydrogen ions to stabilize pH. Whereas the ____________ act immediately, the response by the ____________ may take minutes, and the response in the ____________ much longer.

The four main types of buffer systems are protein, hemoglobin. carbonic acid and bicarbonate, and phosphate.

Regulatory Mechanisms

When the ability of buffer systems is exceeded, acid–base homeostasis is regulated by the lungs and the kidneys.

18. Describe how the following organs adapt to acid–base regulation.

    a. Kidneys: ____

    b. Lungs: ____

Disturbances in electrolyte, fluid, and acid–base balance

Disturbances in electrolyte, fluid, or acid–base balance seldom occur alone and can disrupt normal body processes.

19. The basic types of fluid imbalances include are ____________ and ____________.

20. Isotonic deficit and excess exist when ____________________

21. Osmolar imbalances are ____________________.

22. Complete the grid provided, giving the causes and signs and symptoms of the listed fluid disturbances.

Fluid Disturbances	Causes	Signs and Symptoms
Fluid volume deficit		
Fluid volume excess		
Hyperosmolar imbalance		
Hypoosmolar imbalance		

23. For each electrolyte disturbance, identify the diagnostic laboratory finding, and list at least four characteristic signs and symptoms in the grid provided.

Imbalance	Lab Findings	Signs and Symptoms
Hyponatremia		
Hypernatremia		
Hypokalemia		
Hyperkalemia		
Hypocalcemia		
Hypercalcemia		
Hypomagnesemia		
Hypermagnesemia		

Copyright © 2019 Elsevier Canada, a division of Reed Elsevier Canada, Ltd.

Acid–Base Balance

24. Briefly explain the following components of the acid–base balance.

a. pH:

b. $PaCO_2$:

c. PaO_2:

d. Oxygen saturation:

e. Base excess:

f. Bicarbonate:

Types of acid–base imbalances

25. The four primary types of acid–base imbalances are listed in the following grid. For each acid–base imbalance, identify the diagnostic laboratory finding, and list the characteristic signs and symptoms.

Acid–Base Imbalance	Causes	Signs and Symptoms
Respiratory acidosis		
Respiratory alkalosis		
Metabolic acidosis		
Metabolic alkalosis		

Knowledge Base of Nursing Practice

26. List five major risk factors that can affect fluid and electrolyte imbalances. Give two examples of each.

a.

b.

c.

d.

e.

Assessment

Health history

Age

27. Briefly describe the fluid changes that are associated with aging and development.

a. Infants:

b. Children:

c. Adolescents:

d. Older persons:

Environmental Factors

28. Briefly explain how the following affect fluid, electrolyte, and acid–base imbalances.

a. Environmental factors:

b. Diet:

Copyright © 2019 Elsevier Canada, a division of Reed Elsevier Canada, Ltd.

c. Lifestyle:

d. Medication:

Prior medical history

Acute Illness

29. Explain how the following acute illnesses affect fluid, electrolyte, and acid–base balances.

a. Burns:

b. Respiratory disorders:

c. GI disturbances:

d. Trauma:

e. Head injury:

f. Recent surgery:

Chronic Illness

30. Describe how the following chronic illnesses affect fluid, electrolyte, and acid–base imbalances.

a. Cancer:

b. Cardiovascular disease:

c. Renal disorders:

d. GI disorders:

Physical assessment

A thorough physical examination is necessary because fluid and electrolyte imbalances or acid–base disturbances can affect all body systems.

31. Indicate the possible fluid, electrolyte, or acid–base imbalances associated with each physical finding.

a. Weight changes from previous day:
Loss of 1 kg or more in 24 hours (adults):

Gain of 1 kg or more in 24 hours (adults):

b. Blood pressure:

c. Pulse rate and character:

d. Fullness of neck veins (full and flat):

e. Capillary refill:

f. Lung auscultation:

g. Urine output:

Copyright © 2019 Elsevier Canada, a division of Reed Elsevier Canada, Ltd.

h. Presence of edema: ______________________

i. Mucous membranes: ______________________

j. Skin turgor: ______________________

k. Presence of thirst: ______________________

l. Behaviour and level of consciousness:

Restlessness/mild confusion: ______________________

Decreased level of consciousness: ______________________

m. Pulse rhythm and ECG: ______________________

n. Rate and depth of respirations: ______________________

o. Muscle strength/weakness: ______________________

p. Reflexes and sensations:

Decreased deep tendon reflexes: ______________________

Hyperactive reflexes/muscle twitching and cramps: ______________________

Numbness, tingling in fingertips/mouth: ______________________

Muscle cramps/tetany: ______________________

Tremors: ______________________

q. Abdominal distension: ______________________

r. Decreased bowel sounds: ______________________

s. Motility/constipation: ______________________

Assessing Fluid Intake and Output

32. When implementing specific measures to increase or decrease fluid, three interventions are necessary. Explain each one.

a. Daily weights: ______________________

b. Intake: ______________________

c. Output: ______________________

Recording intake and output is essential for obtaining an accurate database. This information helps maintain an ongoing evaluation of the patient's hydration status to prevent severe imbalances.

Arterial Blood Gases

To determine arterial blood gas levels, a sample of blood from an artery must be taken to assess the patient's acid–base status and the adequacy of ventilation and oxygenation.

Nursing Diagnosis

33. List five potential or actual nursing diagnoses for a patient with fluid, electrolyte, or acid–base imbalances.

a. ______________________

b. ______________________

c. ______________________

d. ______________________

e. ______________________

Copyright © 2019 Elsevier Canada, a division of Reed Elsevier Canada, Ltd.

Planning

Goals and outcomes

34. List three goals that are appropriate for a patient with a fluid, electrolyte, or acid–base imbalance.

a. ____

b. ____

c. ____

Setting priorities

The patient's clinical condition will determine which diagnosis takes the greatest priority. Many nursing diagnoses in the area of fluid, electrolyte, and acid–base balances are of highest priority because the consequences for the patient can be serious or even life threatening.

Implementation

Health promotion

35. Identify some common risk factors for imbalances for which the caregiver may implement appropriate preventive measures.

____

Acute care

Enteral Replacement of Fluids

36. List and briefly describe the enteral replacement of fluids.

a. ____

b. ____

Restriction of Fluids

37. Briefly explain the need for a restricted fluid intake and how the nurse would implement the restriction.

____

Interventions for Acid–Base Imbalances

Nursing interventions to promote acid–base balance support prescribed medical therapies and are aimed at reversing the acid–base imbalance.

Parenteral Replacement of Fluids and Electrolytes

Fluid and electrolytes may be replaced through infusion directly into the blood rather than via the digestive system.

38. List the three methods of parenteral fluid replacement.

a. ____

b. ____

c. ____

39. Total parenteral nutrition is ____.

Vascular Access Devices

40. Vascular access devices are ____.

41. Discuss the difference between peripheral vascular access devices and central vascular access devices.

____

Administration of Intravenous Therapy

42. Identify the primary goal of intravenous (IV) fluid administration.

____

43. Define the following types of electrolyte solutions.

a. Isotonic: ____

b. Hypertonic: ____

c. Hypotonic: ____

Venipuncture Site

44. List three groups of patients for whom venipunctures may be difficult.

a. ____

b. ____

c. ____

Regulating the Infusion Flow Rate

45. List two major purposes of infusion pumps.

a. ____

b. ____

Copyright © 2019 Elsevier Canada, a division of Reed Elsevier Canada, Ltd.

46. List four factors that may affect IV flow rates.
   a. ______
   b. ______
   c. ______
   d. ______

Maintaining the System

47. After the IV line is in place and the flow rate is regulated, you must maintain the system. Line maintenance is achieved by ______, and ______, ______.

Complications of Intravenous Therapy

48. Complete the grid provided, describing complications of IV therapy.

Complication	Assessment Finding	Nursing Action
Infiltration		
Phlebitis		
Bleeding		

Discontinuing Intravenous Infusions

49. Briefly summarize the procedure for discontinuing IV infusions.

Blood Replacement

50. List three objectives for blood transfusion.
   a. ______
   b. ______
   c. ______

Blood Groups and Types

51. Complete the grid provided, describing the ABO compatibilities for major blood groups.

	Donor			
	A	B	O	AB
Recipient of packed red cells (stored, washed, or frozen/washed)				
Recipient of fresh-frozen plasma				
Recipient of platelets				

52. Define a *transfusion reaction.*

Autologous Transfusion

53. Define *autologous transfusion* (autotransfusion).

Blood Transfusions

54. Identify the six nursing interventions associated with blood transfusions and give the rationale for each.
   a. ______
   b. ______
   c. ______
   d. ______
   e. ______
   f. ______

Transfusion Reactions and Complications

A *transfusion reaction* is a systemic response by the body to incompatible blood.

55. Discuss causes of transfusion reactions.

56. Identify types of transfusion reactions and their causes.
   a. ______
   b. ______
   c. ______
   d. ______
   e. ______
   f. ______

Copyright © 2019 Elsevier Canada, a division of Reed Elsevier Canada, Ltd.

57. List the steps the nurse should follow if a transfusion reaction is suspected.
    a. ______
    b. ______
    c. ______
    d. ______
    e. ______
    f. ______
    g. ______
    h. ______

Restorative care

58. Older persons and patients with chronic illnesses require special considerations to prevent complications from developing. Briefly summarize the following considerations.
    a. Home IV therapy:
    ______
    b. Nutritional support:
    ______
    c. Medication safety:
    ______

Evaluation

Patient care

The nurse evaluates the actual care delivered by the health care team based on the expected outcomes.

The nurse will perform evaluative measures and determine if changes have occurred since the last patient assessment. The patient's level of progress determines whether the nurse needs to continue or revise the care plan.

Patient expectations

Nurses routinely review with their patient their success in meeting expectations of care.

Often the patient's level of satisfaction with care also depends on the nurse's success in involving friends and family.

REVIEW QUESTIONS

Select the appropriate answer, and cite the rationale for choosing that particular answer.

1. What are the body fluids that compose the interstitial fluid and blood plasma?
   a. Intracellular
   b. Extracellular
   c. Hypotonic
   d. Hypertonic

Answer: ______ Rationale: ______

2. Which of the following statements is true with regard to the lungs' regulation of acid–base balance?
   a. The lungs serve a minor role in the physiologic buffering of H^+ ions.
   b. It takes several days for the lungs to restore pH to a normal level.
   c. The lungs correct imbalances by altering the rate and depth of respiration.
   d. The lungs maintain normal pH by either retaining or excreting bicarbonate.

Answer: ______ Rationale: ______

3. Mrs. Singh's arterial blood gas results are as follows: pH 7.32; $PaCO_2$ 52 mm Hg; PaO_2 78 mm Hg; HCO_3^- 24 mmol/L. What would you determine Mrs. Singh's arterial blood gases to be?
   a. Respiratory acidosis
   b. Respiratory alkalosis
   c. Metabolic acidosis
   d. Metabolic alkalosis

Answer: ______ Rationale: ______

4. Mr. Frank is an 82-year-old patient with a 3-day history of vomiting and diarrhea. Which symptom would you expect to find on a physical examination?
   a. Neck vein distension
   b. Crackles in the lungs
   c. Tachycardia
   d. Hypertension

Answer: ______ Rationale: ______

Copyright © 2019 Elsevier Canada, a division of Reed Elsevier Canada, Ltd.

5. Which of the following is most likely to result in respiratory alkalosis?
   a. Fad dieting
   b. Hyperventilation
   c. Chronic alcoholism
   d. Steroid use

Answer:________________ Rationale:______________

____

____

CRITICAL THINKING MODEL FOR NURSING CARE PLAN FOR FLUID, ELECTROLYTE, AND ACID–BASE BALANCES

Imagine that you are the student nurse in the Care Plan on pages 1035–1036 of your text. Complete the *planning* phase of the critical thinking model by writing your answers in the appropriate boxes of the model shown. Think about the following:

- When developing a plan of care, what intellectual and professional standards did you apply?
- In developing Mrs. Topping's plan of care, what knowledge did you apply?
- In what way might your previous experience assist you in developing a plan of care for Mrs. Topping?
- What critical thinking attitudes might have been applied in developing Mrs. Topping's care?
- How will you accomplish your goals?

Copyright © 2019 Elsevier Canada, a division of Reed Elsevier Canada, Ltd.

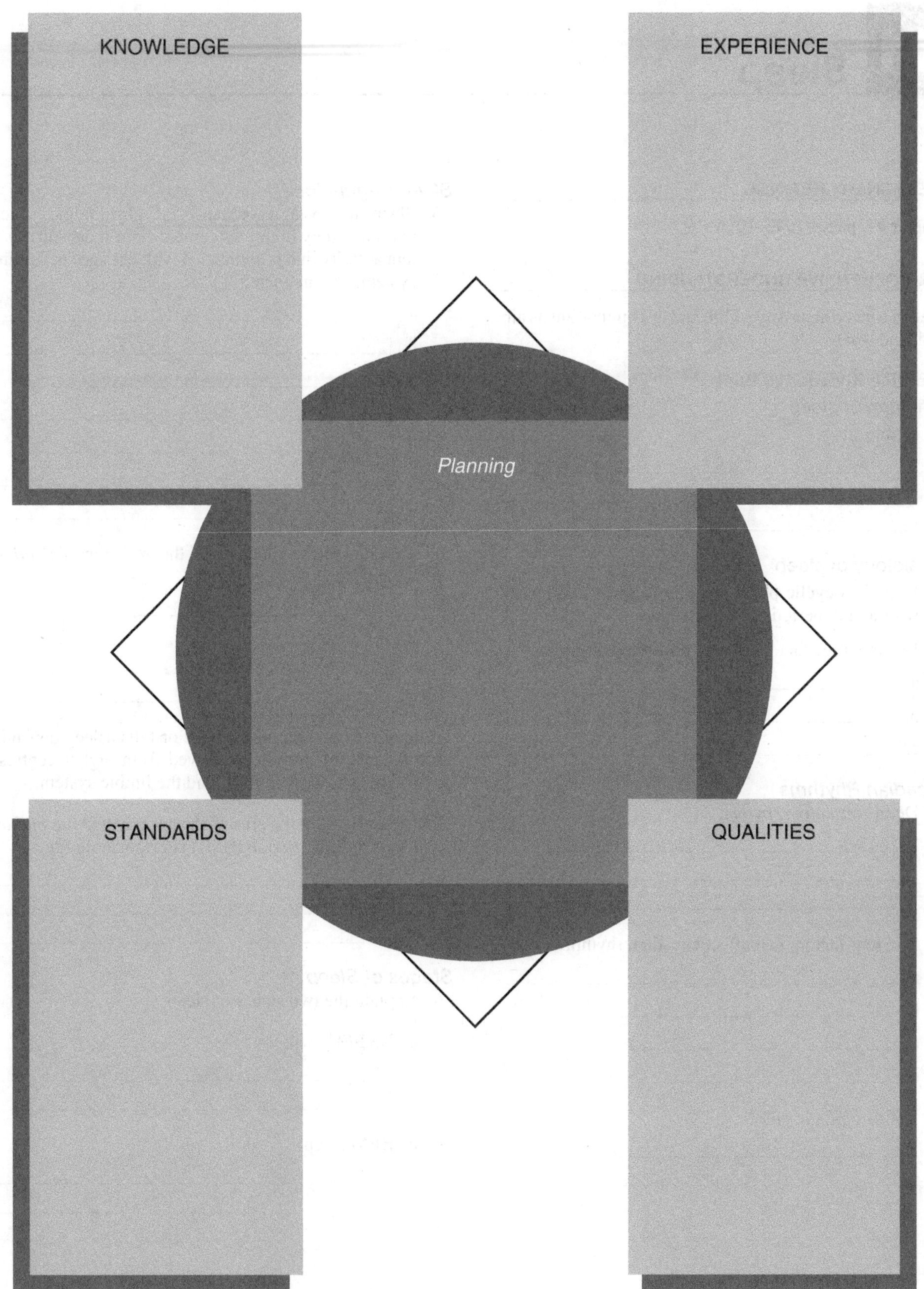

CHAPTER 40 Critical Thinking Model for Nursing Care Plan for *Fluid, Electrolyte, and Acid–Base Balances*
See answers on Evolve site.

Copyright © 2019 Elsevier Canada, a division of Reed Elsevier Canada, Ltd.

41 Sleep

PRELIMINARY READING

Chapter 41, pages 1072–1096

COMPREHENSIVE UNDERSTANDING

Sleep is a basic necessity of life and is as important as air, food, and water.

Scientific Knowledge Base

Definition of sleep

1. Define *sleep.*

____

____

____

Physiology of sleep

2. *Sleep* is a cyclic physiologic process that alternates with longer periods of wakefulness.

   List the three factors that control sleep physiology.

   a. ______________________________

   b. ______________________________

   c. ______________________________

Circadian Rhythms

3. Define *circadian rhythm.*

____

____

____

4. List four factors that affect circadian rhythms.

   a. ______________________________

   b. ______________________________

   c. ______________________________

   d. ______________________________

5. Define *biologic clocks.*

____

____

Sleep Regulation

6. Sleep involves a sequence of physiologic states maintained by highly integrated central nervous system activity that is associated with changes in certain systems. Name them.

   a. ______________________________

   b. ______________________________

   c. ______________________________

   d. ______________________________

   e. ______________________________

   f. ______________________________

   g. ______________________________

7. Summarize the function of the *reticular activating system.*

____

____

____

____

Whether a person remains awake or falls asleep depends on a balance of impulses received from higher centres, peripheral sensory receptors, and the limbic system.

8. Describe what the area of the brain called the *bulbar synchronizing region* (BSR) is responsible for.

____

____

____

Stages of Sleep

9. Explain the two stages of sleep.

   a. NREM sleep:

   ____

   ____

   b. REM sleep:

   ____

   ____

Copyright © 2019 Elsevier Canada, a division of Reed Elsevier Canada, Ltd.

Sleep Cycle

10. Describe the characteristics of the following cycles of sleep.

 a. Stage 1:

 b. Stage 2:

 c. Stage 3:

 d. Stage 4:

 e. REM:

Functions of sleep

11. Explain briefly the functions of sleep.

Dreams

Dreaming is defined as a mental activity that occurs while individuals are asleep.

12. Differentiate between dreams occurring in these two types of sleep.

 a. NREM sleep:

 b. REM sleep:

Physical illness

13. Explain how the following conditions affect sleep.

 a. Illness:

 b. Respiratory disease:

 c. Cardiovascular disease:

 d. Musculoskeletal disorders:

 e. Nocturia:

Sleep disorders

Sleep disorders are conditions that interfere with nighttime sleep. Increasingly, evidence suggests sleep disorders are related to serious medical conditions.

14. Briefly describe the following categories of sleep disorders.

 a. *Hypersomnias*:

 b. *Parasomnias*:

Insomnia

15. Define *insomnia.*

Insomnia is the second most commonly expressed complaint reported in clinical practice after pain. Insomnia is more common in women, and its incidence increases with advancing age.

16. Discuss the condition that is associated with insomnia.

Sleep Apnea

17. Define *sleep apnea.*

Copyright © 2019 Elsevier Canada, a division of Reed Elsevier Canada, Ltd.

18. Define the following types of apnea.

    a. Central sleep apnea:

    ___

    b. Obstructive sleep apnea (OSA):

    ___

19. Discuss the symptoms of OSA.

    ___

20. List the risk factors for developing OSA.

    a. ___
    b. ___
    c. ___
    d. ___
    e. ___
    f. ___
    g. ___

21. Briefly explain excessive daytime sleepiness.

    ___

22. Define *narcolepsy.*

    ___

23. Define *cataplexy.*

    ___

Narcolepsy

24. Identify the developmental stage in which narcolepsy symptoms first develop.

    ___

There is no known cure for narcolepsy; therefore, treatment is targeted at symptom management.

25. Identify the following treatment modalities for a patient with narcolepsy.

    a. Pharmacologic:

    ___

    b. Nonpharmacologic:

    ___

Parasomnias

Parasomnias are undesirable sleep problems that occur while falling asleep, between sleep phases, or during transitions from sleep to wakefulness.

26. Explain the following parasomnias.

    a. Somnambulism:

    ___

    b. Nocturnal enuresis:

    ___

    c. Bruxism:

    ___

Shift Work

Shift work sleep disorder is a common sleep disorder experienced by individuals who work outside the traditional 9-to-5 workday.

27. The most common problems reported by shift workers are ___, ___, and ___, resulting from imposing a sleep–wake schedule that is ___.

Sleep Deprivation

28. Sleep deprivation is ___ ___.

Physicians and nurses are particularly prone to sleep deprivation because of their long work schedules and rotating shifts.

Nursing Knowledge Base

Sleep and rest

29. Define *rest.*

    ___

Copyright © 2019 Elsevier Canada, a division of Reed Elsevier Canada, Ltd.

Normal sleep requirements and patterns

30. Discuss the normal sleep patterns for the various developmental stages listed.

 a. Neonates:

 b. Infants:

 c. Toddlers:

 d. Preschoolers:

 e. School-age children:

 f. Adolescents:

 g. Young adults:

 h. Middle-aged adults:

 i. Older persons:

Factors affecting sleep

31. Sleepiness and sleep deprivation are common side effects of medications. Describe how each of the following affects sleep, and give an example.

 a. Drugs and substances:

 b. Lifestyle:

Usual Sleep Patterns

32. List three alterations in routine that can disrupt sleep patterns.

 a.

 b.

 c.

Emotional Stress

33. Explain how emotional stress affects sleep.

Environment

34. List and briefly describe three environmental factors that affect sleep.

 a.

 b.

 c.

Exercise and Fatigue

35. Explain how exercise promotes sleep.

Food and Caloric Intake

36. List and briefly describe five foods that affect sleep, and why.

 a.

 b.

 c.

 d.

 e.

Nursing Process

Assessment

Sleep and restfulness are subjective experiences. Assessment is aimed at understanding the characteristics of a sleep problem and the patient's sleep habits.

Copyright © 2019 Elsevier Canada, a division of Reed Elsevier Canada, Ltd.

Sleep assessment

Sources for Sleep Assessment

37. Identify three sources for sleep assessment.

a. ______

b. ______

c. ______

Tools for Sleep Assessment

Methods for assessing sleep quality are the use of a visual analogue scale or a numerical scale with a 0-to-10 sleep rating.

Sleep history

38. List seven components of a sleep history.

a. ______

b. ______

c. ______

d. ______

e. ______

f. ______

g. ______

Description of Sleeping Problems

39. List and briefly describe the six areas to assess with a patient when asking about the nature of a sleeping problem.

a. ______

b. ______

c. ______

d. ______

e. ______

f. ______

40. Identify the information recorded in a sleep–wake diary.

______

______

______

______

41. Briefly explain how the following factors interfere with sleep.

a. Physical and psychologic illness:

______

______

______

b. Current life events:

______

______

______

c. Bedtime routines:

______

______

______

d. Bedroom environment:

______

______

______

Behaviours of Sleep Deprivation

42. List four behaviours a patient may manifest with sleep deprivation.

a. ______

b. ______

c. ______

d. ______

Patient expectations

When a patient experiences a poor night's sleep, a vicious cycle of anticipatory anxiety may begin.

Nursing Diagnosis

It is important that your assessment identifies the probable cause of or factors related to the sleep disturbance.

Planning

Goals and outcomes

An effective plan includes outcomes that focus on the goal of improving the quantity and quality of sleep in the home over a realistic period of time.

43. List four goals appropriate for a patient needing rest or sleep.

a. ______

b. ______

c. ______

d. ______

Implementation

Nursing interventions designed to improve the quality of a person's sleep are largely focused on health promotion.

Copyright © 2019 Elsevier Canada, a division of Reed Elsevier Canada, Ltd.

Health promotion

44. Many factors affect the ability to gain adequate rest and sleep. Briefly give examples of each of the following:

   a. Environmental controls:

   b. Promoting bedtime routines:

   c. Promoting safety:

   d. Promoting comfort:

   e. Periods of rest and sleep:

   f. Stress reduction:

   g. Bedtime snacks:

   h. Pharmacologic approaches:

Acute care

45. For each of the following situations, give two examples of nursing measures that will promote sleep.

   a. Environmental controls:
      i.
      ii.

   b. Promoting comfort:
      i.
      ii.

   c. Establishing periods of rest and sleep:
      i.
      ii.

   d. Promoting safety:
      i.
      ii.

   e. Stress reduction:
      i.
      ii.

Restorative or continuing care

46. Give an example of the following interventions that are implemented in the restorative environment.

   a. Promoting comfort:

   b. Controlling physiologic disturbances:

   c. Pharmacologic approaches:

Pharmacological Approaches

47. Briefly describe the effect of benzodiazepines in promoting sleep.

48. Identify three types of patients who should not use benzodiazepines.
   a.
   b.
   c.

49. The regular use of sleep medication can lead to ________.

Evaluation

Each patient has a unique need for sleep and rest, and only the patient will know whether sleep problems have improved and which interventions or therapies are most successful in promoting sleep.

50. Identify some subtle behaviours a patient may exhibit that indicate sleep satisfaction.

Copyright © 2019 Elsevier Canada, a division of Reed Elsevier Canada, Ltd.

REVIEW QUESTIONS

Select the appropriate answer, and cite the rationale for choosing that particular answer.

1. What is the 24-hour day–night cycle known as?
   a. Circadian rhythm
   b. Infradium rhythm
   c. Ultradian rhythm
   d. Non-REM rhythm

Answer: ______________ Rationale: ______________

____

____

2. Which of the following substances will promote normal sleep patterns?
   a. L-tryptophan
   b. Beta-adrenergic blockers
   c. Alcohol
   d. Narcotics

Answer: ______________ Rationale: ______________

____

____

3. Which of the following is not a symptom of sleep deprivation?
   a. Hyperactivity
   b. Irritability
   c. Rise in body temperature
   d. Decreased motivation

Answer: ______________ Rationale: ______________

____

____

4. Mrs. Phan complains of difficulty falling asleep, awakening earlier than desired, and not feeling rested. She attributes these problems to leg pain that is secondary to her arthritis. What would be the appropriate nursing diagnosis for her?
   a. Sleep pattern disturbances related to arthritis
   b. Fatigue related to leg pain
   c. Knowledge deficit related to sleep hygiene measures
   d. Sleep pattern disturbances related to chronic leg pain

Answer: ______________ Rationale: ______________

____

____

5. A nursing care plan for a patient with sleep problems has been implemented. Which of the following would *not* be an expected outcome?
   a. Patient reports no episodes of awakening during the night.
   b. Patient falls asleep within 1 hour of going to bed.
   c. Patient reports satisfaction with amount of sleep.
   d. Patient rates sleep as an 8 or above on the visual analogue scale.

Answer: ______________ Rationale: ______________

____

____

CRITICAL THINKING MODEL FOR NURSING CARE PLAN FOR DISTURBED SLEEP PATTERN

Imagine that you are the nurse in the Care Plan on pages 1087–1088 of your text. Complete the *evaluation* phase of the critical thinking model by writing your answers in the appropriate boxes of the model shown. Think about the following:

- What knowledge did you apply in evaluating Andree's care?
- In what way might your previous experience influence your evaluation of Andree's care?
- During evaluation, what intellectual and professional standards were applied to Andree's care?
- In what way do critical thinking attitudes play a role in how you approach the evaluation of Julie's care plan?
- How might you evaluate Andree's care plan?

Copyright © 2019 Elsevier Canada, a division of Reed Elsevier Canada, Ltd.

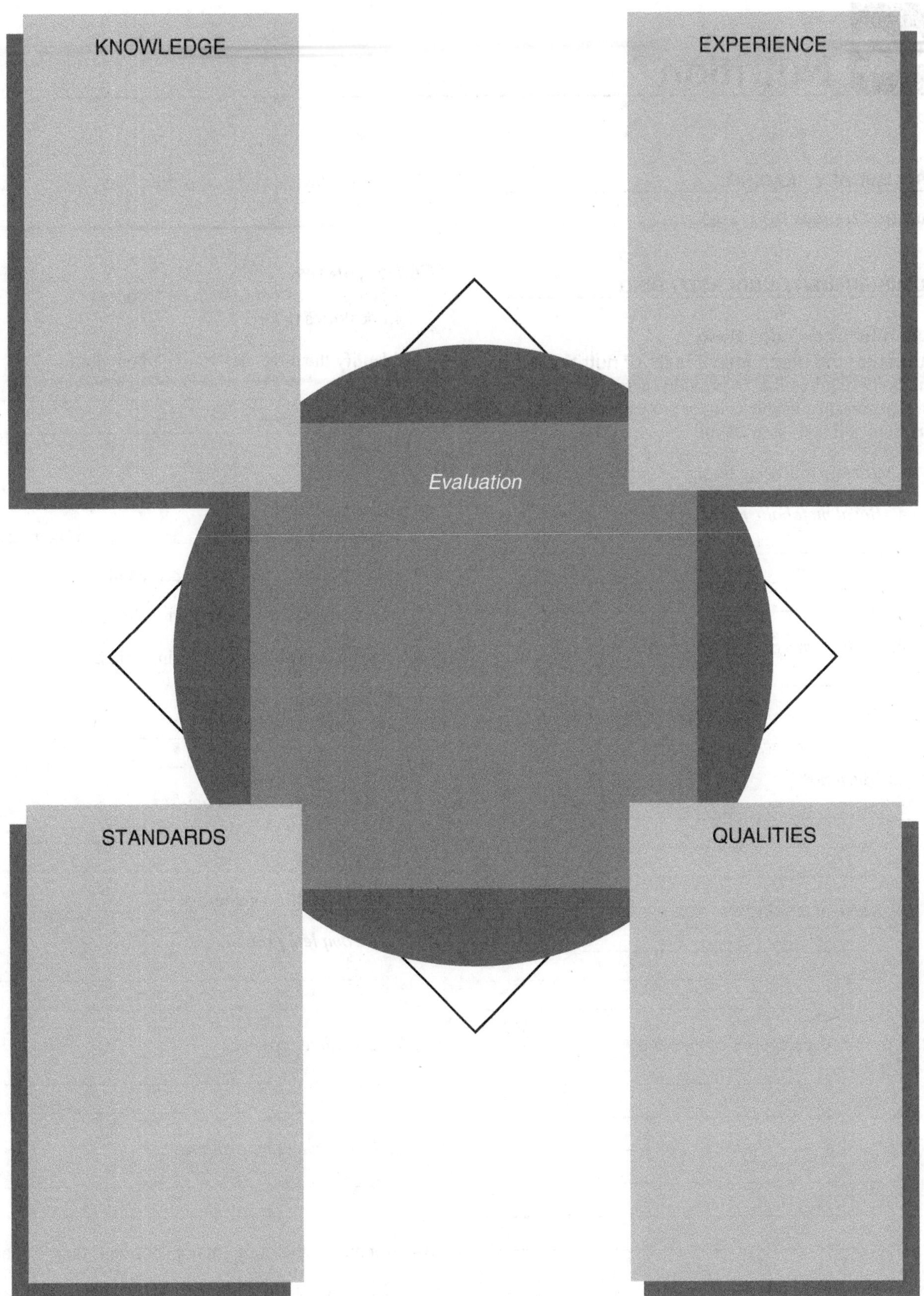

CHAPTER 41 Critical Thinking Model for Nursing Care Plan for *Disturbed Sleep Pattern*
See answers on Evolve site.

Copyright © 2019 Elsevier Canada, a division of Reed Elsevier Canada, Ltd.

42 Nutrition

PRELIMINARY READING

Chapter 42, pages 1097–1165

COMPREHENSIVE UNDERSTANDING

Scientific Knowledge Base

Nutrients: the biochemical units of nutrition

The body requires fuel to provide energy for the chemical reactions that enable cellular growth and repair, organ function, and body movement.

1. Define the following terms.
   a. *Basal metabolic rate*:
   ____
   ____
   ____
   b. *Resting energy expenditure*:
   ____
   ____
   ____
   c. *Nutrients*:
   ____
   ____
   ____
   d. *Nutrient density*:
   ____
   ____
   ____
2. List the six categories of nutrients.
   a. ______________________
   b. ______________________
   c. ______________________
   d. ______________________
   e. ______________________
   f. ______________________
3. Foods may also be described as __________, __________, or __________.

Carbohydrates

4. Each gram of *carbohydrate* produces __________ kilocalories (kcal).
5. Identify the three classes of carbohydrates.
   a. ______________________
   b. ______________________
   c. ______________________

Proteins

6. Proteins are essential for __________ of body tissue in __________, __________, and __________.
7. The simplest form of protein is the __________.
8. Explain the two types of amino acids.
   a. *Essential amino acids*:
   ____
   ____
   b. *Nonessential amino acids*:
   ____
   ____
9. Define the following terms.
   a. *Incomplete protein*:
   ____
   ____
   b. *Complete protein*:
   ____
   ____
   c. *Complementary proteins*:
   ____
   ____
10. Protein is the only major nutrient that contains __________ and is the only source of __________ for the body.

Copyright © 2019 Elsevier Canada, a division of Reed Elsevier Canada, Ltd.

11. *Nitrogen balance* is ______________________________
______________________________.

Fats

12. Fats (*lipids*) are the most calorically dense nutrient, providing __________ kcal/g.

13. Describe the composition of the following forms of fats.

    a. Triglycerides:
    ____
    ____

    b. Fatty acids:
    ____
    ____

14. Define the following types of fatty acids, and give an example of each.

    a. Saturated fatty acids:
    ____
    ____

    b. Unsaturated fatty acids:
    ____
    ____

    c. Monounsaturated fatty acids:
    ____
    ____

    d. Polyunsaturated fatty acids:
    ____
    ____

    e. Trans fatty acids:
    ____
    ____

15. Define *cholesterol*, and identify two sources of cholesterol.
____
____
____
____

Water

16. Water makes up __________ of total body weight.

17. __________ have the greatest percentage of total body weight as water, and __________ have the least.

18. Fluid needs are met by ingesting __________ and __________, and by water produced during ______________________________.

19. Identify the role of water in the body.
____
____
____
____

Vitamins

20. *Vitamins* are ______________________________
______________________________.

21. Identify the *fat-soluble vitamins*.

    a. ______________________________
    b. ______________________________
    c. ______________________________
    d. ______________________________

22. Identify the *water-soluble vitamins*:

    a. ______________________________
    b. ______________________________

23. Define *hypervitaminosis*.
____
____
____
____

Minerals

24. *Minerals* are ______________________________.

25. Minerals are classified as __________ when the daily requirement is 100 mg or more, and as __________ or __________ when fewer than 100 mg are needed daily.

Anatomy and physiology of the digestive system

Digestion

Digestion of food consists of the mechanical breakdown and chemical reactions by which food is reduced to its simplest form.

Copyright © 2019 Elsevier Canada, a division of Reed Elsevier Canada, Ltd.

26. *Enzymes* are ______________________________.

27. Explain the mechanical, chemical, and hormonal activities of digestion.

____

____

28. The major portion of digestion occurs in the ______________________________.

29. Define the following terms.

a. *Peristalsis*:

____

____

b. *Chyme*:

____

____

Absorption

30. The primary absorption site of nutrients is the ______________________________.

31. The main source of water absorption is via the ______________________________.

32. In addition to water, electrolytes and minerals are absorbed, and bacteria in the colon synthesize vitamin __________ and some ______________________.

Metabolism and Storage of Nutrients

33. *Metabolism* refers to ______________________________.

34. Describe the two types of metabolism.

a. Anabolism:

____

____

b. Catabolism:

____

____

35. *Nutrient metabolism* consists of three main processes. Explain each one.

a. Glycogenolysis:

____

____

b. Glycogenesis:

____

____

c. Gluconeogenesis:

____

____

36. Glycogen is synthesized from ______________________________.

37. The body's major form of reserved energy is __________, which is stored as ______________.

Elimination

38. Feces contain ______________________________.

Dietary guidelines

Dietary Reference Intakes

39. Explain *dietary reference intakes.*

____

____

____

____

40. Define the four components to the dietary reference intakes.

a. ______________________________

b. ______________________________

c. ______________________________

d. ______________________________

Copyright © 2019 Elsevier Canada, a division of Reed Elsevier Canada, Ltd.

Food Guidelines

41. Using the space provided, diagram and label *Canada's Food Guide.*

42. List five dietary guidelines identified in *Eating Well With Canada's Food Guide.*

a. ___

b. ___

c. ___

d. ___

e. ___

43. List the nutritional recommendations identified in *Eating Well With Canada's Food Guide.*

a. ___

b. ___

c. ___

d. ___

e. ___

f. ___

g. ___

h. ___

Copyright © 2019 Elsevier Canada, a division of Reed Elsevier Canada, Ltd.

Nursing Knowledge Base

Nutrition during human growth and development

Infants Through School-Age Children

44. An energy intake of approximately ________ kcal/kg is needed in the first half of infancy, and ________ kcal/kg is needed in the second half of infancy.

45. A full-term newborn is able to digest and absorb ________, ________, and ________.

46. Infants need ________ mL/kg per day of fluid.

Breastfeeding

47. List at least four benefits for breastfeeding an infant.

a. ________
b. ________
c. ________
d. ________

Formula

48. Explain why the following should not be used in infant formula.

a. Cow's milk:

____

b. Honey:

____

Introduction to Solid Food

49. The addition of solid foods to an infant's diet should be governed by the infant's:

a. ________
b. ________
c. ________
d. ________
e. ________
f. ________

50. When should dental visits begin?

____

51. What practice puts children at risk for developing early-childhood tooth decay? Why?

____

52. What is the role of parents in ensuring the dental health of their young child?

____

53. The toddler needs ________ kilocalories, but an increased amount of ________ in relation to body weight.

54. Identify examples of foods that have been implicated in the choking deaths of toddlers and preschoolers.

____

55. School-age children's diets should be assessed for ________.

56. Explain some reasons for the increase in childhood obesity.

____

Adolescents

57. Identify the common nutritional deficiencies in the following adolescent population groups.

a. Girls:

____

b. Boys:

____

c. Those who eat fast food:

____

Copyright © 2019 Elsevier Canada, a division of Reed Elsevier Canada, Ltd.

d. Athletes:

______

______

______

e. Pregnant adolescent girls aged 14 to 18:

______

______

______

58. Identify the diagnostic criteria for the following eating disorders.

a. *Anorexia nervosa*:

______

______

b. *Bulimia nervosa*:

______

______

Young and Middle-Aged Adults

59. Obesity may become a problem because of ______.

60. Adult women who use oral contraceptives need extra ______.

Pregnancy

61. The energy requirements of pregnancy are related to ______ and ______.

62. During pregnancy, supplementation is usually recommended along with dietary modification to increase intake of the following:

a. ______

b. ______

c. ______

Lactation

63. During lactation, there is an increased need for vitamins ______ and ______.

Older Persons

64. List four factors that influence the nutritional status of the older person.

a. ______

b. ______

c. ______

d. ______

Alternative food patterns

Vegetarian Diet

65. What knowledge is necessary to implement a healthy vegetarian diet?

______

______

______

______

Nursing Process and Nutrition

Close daily contact with patients and their families enables nurses to make observations about their physical status, food intake, weight changes, and responses to therapy.

Assessment

66. Define the following terms.

a. *Nutritional screening*:

______

______

______

b. *Nutritional assessment*:

______

______

______

c. *Anthropometry*:

______

______

______

d. *Ideal body weight*:

______

______

______

e. *Body mass index*:

______

______

______

67. Describe how to obtain a *waist circumference* measurement.

______

______

______

______

Copyright © 2019 Elsevier Canada, a division of Reed Elsevier Canada, Ltd.

Laboratory and biochemical tests

68. Identify the common laboratory tests used to study the nutritional status of a patient.

Dietary history and health history

69. List 12 components of a dietary history, and provide a sample question for each.
    a.
    b.
    c.
    d.
    e.
    f.
    g.
    h.
    i.
    j.
    k.
    l.

Clinical observation and physical examination

70. For each assessment area, list at least two signs of good and poor nutrition.
    a. General appearance:
    b. General vitality:
    c. Weight:
    d. Hair:
    e. Skin:
    f. Mouth, oral membranes:
    g. GI function:
    h. Cardiovascular function:
    i. Nervous system function:
    j. Muscles:

71. Define the following terms.
    a. *Aspiration*:
    b. *Dysphagia*:

72. Describe the steps involved in an in-depth assessment for aspiration risk.

73. Identify the warning signs of dysphagia.

Nursing Diagnosis

74. List three potential or actual nursing diagnoses for altered nutritional status.
    a.
    b.
    c.

Copyright © 2019 Elsevier Canada, a division of Reed Elsevier Canada, Ltd.

Planning

The planning for enhanced, optimal nutritional status requires a higher level of care than simply correcting problems. Information from multiple sources must be synthesized to devise an individualized approach to care that is relevant to the patient's needs.

Goals and outcomes

75. Provide an example of a goal and associated outcomes appropriate for a patient with nutritional problems.

    Goal: ______

    Outcomes: ______

    a. ______
    b. ______
    c. ______
    d. ______

Implementation

Health promotion/illness prevention

76. Nurses are in a key position to educate patients about ______.

77. Describe the relationship between income and healthy eating.

78. List two examples of interventions to counter the threat to nutrition and health from lack of purchasing power.

    a. Individual level:

    b. Collective level:

79. Patient education about food safety and reducing the risk of foodborne illnesses includes the following instructions.

    a. ______
    b. ______
    c. ______
    d. ______
    e. ______
    f. ______
    g. ______
    h. ______
    i. ______
    j. ______

Acute care

80. List three factors that can cause *anorexia* (loss of appetite) in acute care settings.

    a. ______
    b. ______
    c. ______

81. Identify factors that put patients at nutritional risk during hospitalizations.

82. Describe the following therapeutic diets.

    a. Clear liquid:

    b. Thickened liquid:

    c. Full liquid:

    d. Puréed:

    e. Mechanical soft:

    f. Soft or low residue:

    g. High fibre:

Copyright © 2019 Elsevier Canada, a division of Reed Elsevier Canada, Ltd.

h. Low sodium:

i. Low cholesterol:

j. Diabetic:

k. Regular:

Promoting Appetite

83. List five ways in which you can promote appetite.
   a.
   b.
   c.
   d.
   e.

Assisting patients with feeding

84. List eight nursing interventions to assist dysphagic patients with feeding.
   a.
   b.
   c.
   d.
   e.
   f.
   g.
   h.

85. List six nursing measures to help patients retain comfort and a sense of independence in relation to their food intake.
   a.
   b.
   c.
   d.
   e.
   f.

Evaluation

Patient care

Patient Expectations

86. Patients expect competent and accurate care. You must ________ if outcomes of nutritional therapies are unsuccessful.

Self-Monitoring of Blood Glucose

87. By providing a real-time blood glucose reading, self-monitoring of blood glucose enables the patient to make self-management decisions regarding diet, exercise, and medication ________.

88. The frequency of monitoring blood sugar depends on:
   a.
   b.
   c.
   d.

Enteral Tube Feeding

89. Briefly describe *enteral nutrition.*

Preventing complications

90. Risks of complications associated with enteral feedings are increased with:
   a.
   b.
   c.
   d.
   e.

91. Discuss the major complications of enteral nutrition.

Large-Bore Tube and Nasogastric or Orogastric Suctioning

92. Discuss *gastric decompression.*

Parenteral Nutrition

93. Define *parental nutrition.*

Copyright © 2019 Elsevier Canada, a division of Reed Elsevier Canada, Ltd.

Preventing complications

94. Discuss 10 complications of parenteral nutrition.

REVIEW QUESTIONS

Select the appropriate answer, and cite the rationale for choosing that particular answer.

1. Which nutrient is the body's preferred energy source?
   a. Protein
   b. Fat
   c. Carbohydrate
   d. Vitamins

Answer:________ Rationale:________

2. In which condition does a positive nitrogen balance occur?
   a. Infection
   b. Starvation
   c. Burn injury
   d. Wound healing

Answer:________ Rationale:________

3. Mrs. Schultz is talking with you about the dietary needs of her 23-month-old daughter, Anita. Which of the following responses would be appropriate?
   a. "Use skim milk to cut down on the fat in Anita's diet."
   b. "Anita should be drinking at least 720 mL of milk per day."
   c. "Anita needs fewer calories in relation to her body weight now than she did as an infant."
   d. "Anita needs less protein in her diet now because she isn't growing as fast."

Answer:________ Rationale:________

4. Which patient is *not* at risk for alteration in nutrition?
   a. Patient J, who is 86 years old, lives alone, and has poorly fitting dentures
   b. Patient K, who has been on nothing-by-mouth status for 7 days following bowel surgery and is receiving intravenous fluids
   c. Patient L, whose weight is 10% above his ideal body weight
   d. Patient M, a 17-year-old girl who weighs 40 kg and frequently complains about her baby fat

Answer:________ Rationale:________

5. What is the best recommendation to help 9- to 11-year-olds counter childhood obesity?
   a. Consume two to three servings of fruit and vegetables daily.
   b. Consume two to three servings of milk products daily.
   c. Eliminate all fat from the daily diet.
   d. Reduce the hours spent in front of the television.

Answer:________ Rationale:________

6. Which of the following is often found to be high when analyzing the current diet of Aboriginal peoples?
   a. Calcium
   b. Fibre
   c. Fat and sugar
   d. Fruits and vegetables

Answer:________ Rationale:________

CRITICAL THINKING MODEL FOR NURSING CARE PLAN FOR IMBALANCED NUTRITION: LESS THAN BODY REQUIREMENTS

Imagine that you are Belinda, the nurse in the Care Plan on pages 1121–1122 of your text. Complete the *planning* phase of the critical thinking model by writing your answers in the appropriate boxes of the model shown. Think about the following:

- In developing Mrs. Cooper's plan of care, what knowledge did Belinda apply?
- In what ways might Belinda's previous experience assist in developing Mrs. Cooper's plan of care?
- When developing a plan of care for Mrs. Cooper, what intellectual and professional standards were applied?
- What critical thinking attitudes might have been applied in developing Mrs. Cooper's plan of care?
- How will Belinda accomplish these goals?

Copyright © 2019 Elsevier Canada, a division of Reed Elsevier Canada, Ltd.

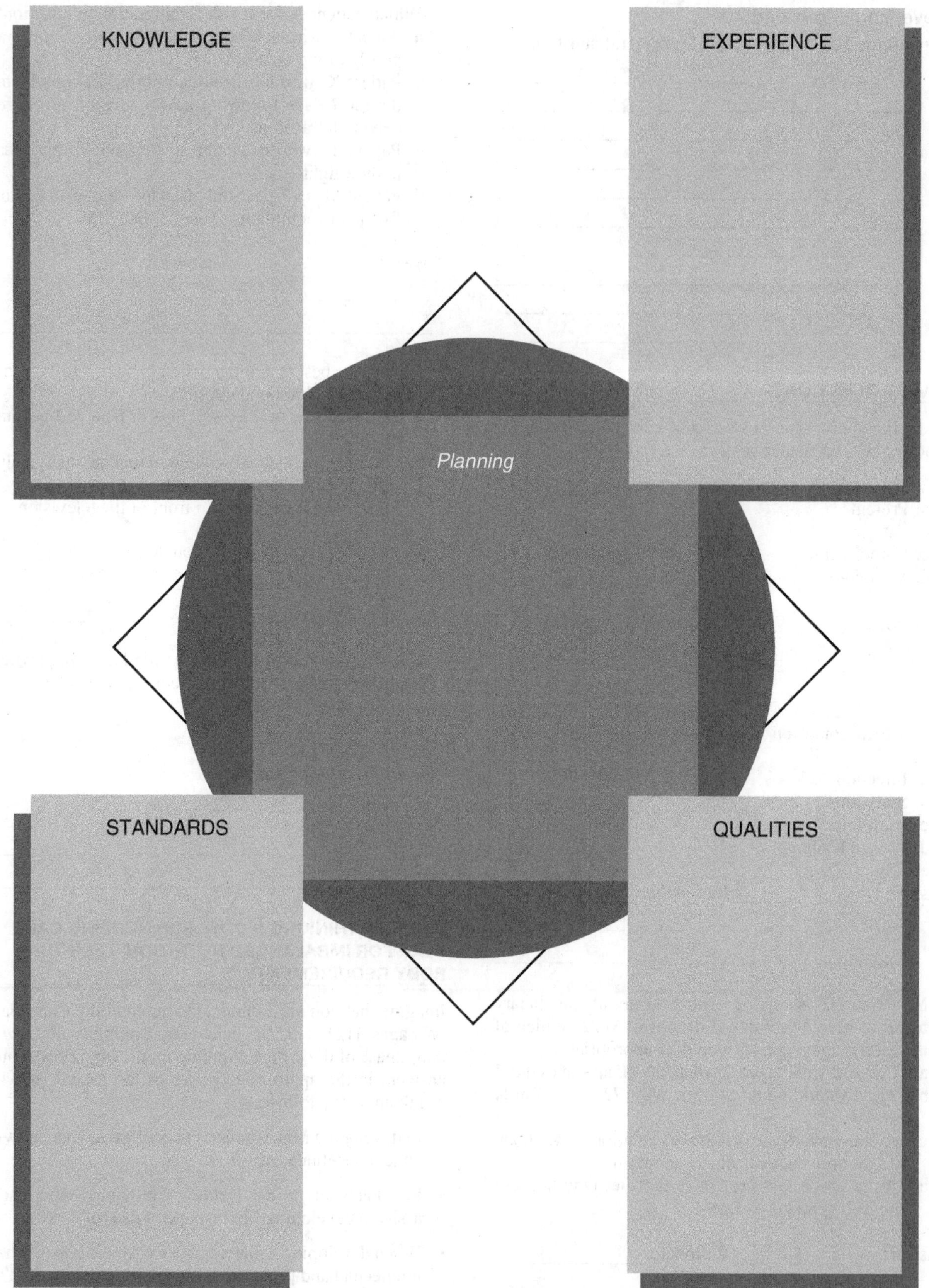

CHAPTER 42 Critical Thinking Model for Nursing Care Plan for *Imbalanced Nutrition: Less Than Body Requirements*
See answers on Evolve site.

Copyright © 2019 Elsevier Canada, a division of Reed Elsevier Canada, Ltd.

43 Urinary Elimination

PRELIMINARY READING

Chapter 43, pages 1166–1210

COMPREHENSIVE UNDERSTANDING

Scientific Knowledge Base

1. Summarize the function of each of the following organs in the urinary system.

   a. Kidneys:

   b. Ureters:

   c. Bladder:

   d. Urethra:

2. Define the following terms related to urine elimination.

   a. *Nephron*:

   b. *Proteinuria*:

   c. *Erythropoietin*:

   d. *Renin*:

   e. *Micturition*:

   f. *Urethral meatus*:

The ability of the urethra to maintain adequate closure is critical to continence.

3. Briefly describe the *urethral closure mechanism.*

Act of urination

4. Number the steps describing the normal act of *micturition* in sequential order.

   _____ The detrusor muscle contracts.

   _____ Sensory nerves from the bladder and urethra carry efferent signals through the reflex arc, sending impulses to the micturition centre in the spinal cord.

   _____ The urethral sphincter relaxes.

   _____ Impulses travel up from the pontine micturition centre.

   _____ The bladder empties.

Factors influencing urination

Pathophysiologic conditions may be acute and reversible (urinary tract infection, or UTI), whereas others may be chronic and irreversible (slow, progressive development of renal dysfunction).

Psychologic Factors

5. __________ and __________ may cause a sense of urgency and increased__________. __________ also may prevent a person from being able to __________ completely; as a result, the urge to void may return __________.

Fluid Balance

6. Explain how the following factors affect the balance of urine excreted.

   a. Caffeine drinks:

Copyright © 2019 Elsevier Canada, a division of Reed Elsevier Canada, Ltd.

b. Alcohol:

Diagnostic Examination

7. Explain what *cystoscopy* is and how it may affect urination.

Surgical Procedures

8. Briefly explain how the stress of surgery affects urine output.

Pathologic Conditions

9. Discuss how each of the following conditions can affect urinary elimination.

a. Central nervous system:

b. Neurologic disease:

c. Spinal cord injury:

d. Advanced dementia:

e. Slow or hindered mobility:

f. Urine volume and quantity:

Medications

10. List three types of medications that affect urination, and describe their major effect.

a.

b.

c.

11. Disease processes that primarily affect renal function (changes in urine volume or quality) are generally categorized as follows. Briefly explain each.

a. Prerenal:

b. Renal:

c. Postrenal:

Common alterations in urinary elimination

12. Most patients with urinary problems have disturbances in the act of micturition that involve a failure to store urine, a failure to empty urine, or both. List the four most common alterations in urinary elimination.

a.

b.

c.

d.

Urinary Tract Infections

13. Although several microorganisms may cause UTIs, __________ is the most frequent causative pathogen.

14. Describe two host defence mechanisms specific to each of the following groups.

a. Both females and males:

b. Females:

c. Males:

Copyright © 2019 Elsevier Canada, a division of Reed Elsevier Canada, Ltd.

15. List four risk factors for UTI in women.
    a. ____
    b. ____
    c. ____
    d. ____

16. Identify the most common cause of UTIs.

____

Signs and Symptoms

17. List six signs or symptoms of UTIs.
    a. ____
    b. ____
    c. ____
    d. ____
    e. ____
    f. ____

18. Define the following terms related to UTIs.
    a. *Pyelonephritis*:
    b. *Bacteriuria*:

19. Explain why residual urine is a risk factor for UTIs.

____.

20. Define *urinary incontinence.*

Overactive Bladder Syndrome

21. Explain the term *overactive bladder*.

22. Briefly describe the major types of urinary incontinence.
    a. Transient:
    b. Urgency:
    c. Stress:
    d. Mixed:
    e. Associated with chronic retention of urine:
    f. Functional:

Nocturia

Nocturia has been defined as waking at night to void. It is associated with aging and an overactive bladder, as well as with an enlarged prostate in men.

Urinary Retention

23. Define *urinary retention.*

24. List five signs of urinary retention.
    a. ____
    b. ____
    c. ____
    d. ____
    e. ____

Urinary Diversions

25. Identify three indications for urinary diversions.
    a. ____
    b. ____
    c. ____

26. Briefly describe the following urinary diversions.
    a. Ileal loop or conduit:

Copyright © 2019 Elsevier Canada, a division of Reed Elsevier Canada, Ltd.

b. Ureterostomy:

c. Nephrostomy:

27. List the characteristic signs of the *uremic syndrome.*

Renal Replacement Therapies

28. Briefly describe the two methods of dialysis.

a. Peritoneal dialysis:

b. Hemodialysis:

29. Identify some indications for dialysis.

Nursing Knowledge Base

You need to know concepts other than anatomy and physiology, as well as an understanding of concepts such as infection control, hygiene measures, growth and development, and psychosocial influences.

Infection control and hygiene

30. Hospital-acquired UTIs are often related to ______, ______, or ______.

Growth and development

31. Briefly summarize the developmental changes that may influence urination.

Psychosocial and cultural considerations

32. Identify the psychosocial and cultural factors that may influence urination.

Nursing Process and Alterations in Urinary Function

Assessment

To identify a urinary elimination problem, obtain information by collecting a health history, performing a focused physical assessment, assessing the patient's urine, and reviewing information from diagnostic tests and examinations.

Health history

33. List three factors to be explored when completing a health history related to urinary elimination.

a. ______

b. ______

c. ______

34. List five topics that should be included in a *urinary diary.*

a. ______

b. ______

c. ______

d. ______

e. ______

Factors Affecting Urination

35. Describe the following symptoms of urinary alterations.

a. Incontinence:

b. Urgency:

c. Dysuria:

d. Frequency:

Copyright © 2019 Elsevier Canada, a division of Reed Elsevier Canada, Ltd.

e. Hesitancy: ____________________

f. Polyuria: ____________________

g. Oliguria: ____________________

h. Nocturia: ____________________

i. Dribbling: ____________________

j. Hematuria: ____________________

k. Elevated postvoid residual urine: ____________________

Physical assessment

36. Briefly explain the four structures assessed in a physical exam to determine the presence and severity of urinary problems.

a. ____________________

b. ____________________

c. ____________________

d. ____________________

Assessment of urine

37. Assessment of urine involves ____________________ and ____________________.

Characteristics of Urine

38. Describe the following characteristics of urine.

a. Colour: ____________________

b. Clarity: ____________________

c. Odour: ____________________

Urine Testing

39. Describe the following types of urine specimens collected for testing.

a. Random: ____________________

b. Clean-voided or midstream: ____________________

c. Catheter: ____________________

d. Timed: ____________________

Common Urine Tests

40. Common urine tests include the following. Briefly explain each.

a. *Urinalysis*: ____________________

b. *Specific gravity*: ____________________

Copyright © 2019 Elsevier Canada, a division of Reed Elsevier Canada, Ltd.

c. *Urine culture*:

Diagnostic examinations

41. Briefly explain the following types of diagnostic examinations, and give the nursing implications for each.

a. Abdominal roentgenogram:

b. Computerized axial tomography scan:

c. Intravenous pyelogram:

d. Renal scan:

e. Ultrasonography:

42. List the three types of invasive diagnostic examinations and the nursing implications.

a.

b.

c.

Nursing Diagnosis

43. List six potential or actual nursing diagnoses related to urinary elimination.

a.

b.

c.

d.

e.

f.

Planning

Goals and outcomes

44. List two examples of goals appropriate for a patient with a urinary elimination problem.

Implementation

Health promotion

45. Identify five health topics that the primary health provider should teach on bladder health.

a.

b.

c.

d.

e.

Promoting Regular Micturition

46. Maintaining regular patterns of urinary elimination can help prevent many urination problems. You should reinforce the importance of voiding regularly every

_____ to _____ hours during the day.

Stimulating Micturition Reflex

47. List three techniques that may be used to stimulate the micturition reflex.

a.

b.

c.

Maintaining Adequate Fluid Intake

48. Maintaining an adequate fluid intake of _____ to _____ mL promotes continence because concentrated urine can irritate the bladder mucosa.

Avoiding Food and Fluids That Can Irritate the Bladder Mucosa

49. List several food substances that can be irritating to the bladder mucosa.

Promoting Complete Bladder Emptying

Normally, a small amount of urine remains in the bladder after voiding; however, urinary incontinence may occur when too much residual urine is in the bladder or when the urinary sphincters are too weak to maintain closure pressure.

Preventing Infection

50. One of the most important considerations for a patient with alterations in urinary elimination is the need to prevent infection of the urinary system. List three preventative measures.

a.

b.

c.

Copyright © 2019 Elsevier Canada, a division of Reed Elsevier Canada, Ltd.

Acute care

Maintaining Elimination Habits

51. Briefly explain how you can help the hospitalized patient to maintain normal elimination habits.

Medications

52. List and explain three types of medications that can be used to treat incontinence or retention.
   a.
   b.
   c.

Catheterization

53. List three indications for each of the following:
   a. Short-term catheterization:
   b. Long-term catheterization:
   c. Intermittent catheterization:

Types of Catheterization

54. Briefly describe the following types of catheters.
   a. Straight:
   b. Coudé:
   c. Foley:

Catheter Insertion

For urethral catheterization of any type, a physician's order is required. You must use the strict aseptic technique.

Routine Catheter Care

55. Explain the following nursing measures taken to maintain patient comfort, prevent infection, and maintain an unobstructed flow of urine in catheterized patients.
   a. Perineal hygiene:
   b. Catheter care:
   c. Fluid intake:

Preventing Infection

The most important strategy in preventing the onset of infection is performing hand hygiene between patients.

Catheter Irrigations and Instillations

56. Briefly describe catheter irrigations and instillations.

Removal of In-Dwelling Catheter

57. Name two benefits of removing an in-dwelling catheter.
   a.
   b.

Alternatives to Urethral Catheterization

58. Briefly explain the two alternatives for urinary catheterization, and give the nursing implications for each.
   a. Suprapubic catheterization:
   b. Condom catheterization:

Copyright © 2019 Elsevier Canada, a division of Reed Elsevier Canada, Ltd.

Maintenance of Skin Integrity

59. List the nursing measures used to maintain skin integrity when urine comes in contact with the skin.
    a. ____________
    b. ____________
    c. ____________
    d. ____________

Promotion of Comfort

60. List comfort measures for a patient with the following sources of discomfort.
    a. Inflamed tissues near urethral meatus: ____________
    b. Painful distension: ____________

Conservative therapies to restore bladder control and promote continence

61. List measures the nurse can teach the incontinent patient to gain control over elimination.
    a. ____________
    b. ____________
    c. ____________
    d. ____________
    e. ____________
    f. ____________
    g. ____________
    h. ____________
    i. ____________
    j. ____________
62. Conservative therapies should be the first line of treatment because they are ____________, have ____________, and ____________.

Lifestyle Modification

63. Describe three lifestyle modifications that can improve symptoms of urinary incontinence.
    a. ____________
    b. ____________
    c. ____________

Pelvic Floor Muscle Exercises

64. Define *pelvic floor muscle (PFM) exercises* (Kegel exercises), and list the types of incontinence for which they are generally indicated.
    ____

Bladder Training

65. Describe a regimen of bladder training and the patients most likely to benefit.
    ____

Habit Retraining and Prompted Voiding

66. Describe the behavioural therapies most appropriate for patients with cognitive impairment, physical impairment, or both.
    a. ____________
    b. ____________

Evaluation

Patient care

The patient is the best source of evaluation of outcomes and responses to nursing care; however, the nurse also evaluates interventions through comparisons with baseline data.

67. You should evaluate for changes in the ____________, ____________, and ____________.

Patient expectations

You need to confirm whether the patient's expectations have been met to his or her full satisfaction.

You can also assist the patient in redefining unrealistic goals when an impairment is not likely to be altered as completely as the patient might like.

Copyright © 2019 Elsevier Canada, a division of Reed Elsevier Canada, Ltd.

REVIEW QUESTIONS

Select the appropriate answer, and cite the rationale for choosing that particular answer.

1. Which factor will *not* influence the production of urine?
   a. Poor PFM tone
   b. Acute renal disease
   c. Febrile conditions
   d. Diuretic medications

Answer: ______________ Rationale: ______________

2. Which term is used to describe a small amount of leaking urine when a female coughs or laughs?
   a. Transient incontinence
   b. Stress incontinence
   c. Urge incontinence
   d. Reflex incontinence

Answer: ______________ Rationale: ______________

3. Ms. Worobetz has a UTI. Which of the following symptoms would you expect her to exhibit?
   a. Proteinuria
   b. Oliguria
   c. Dysuria
   d. Polyuria

Answer: ______________ Rationale: ______________

4. The nurse is working with a patient who is having an intravenous pyelogram. Which of the following complaints by the patient is an abnormal response?
   a. Shortness of breath and audible wheezing
   b. Feeling dizzy and warm with obvious facial flushing
   c. Thirst and feeling "worn out"
   d. Frequent, loose stools

Answer: ______________ Rationale: ______________

5. A postsurgical patient who has recently had her indwelling catheter removed complains of feeling the urge to void every 20 to 30 minutes but is only voiding small amounts. Which of the following behavioural therapies would be most appropriate?
   a. Habit retraining
   b. Prompted voiding
   c. PFM exercise
   d. Bladder training

Answer: ______________ Rationale: ______________

CRITICAL THINKING MODEL FOR NURSING CARE PLAN FOR FUNCTIONAL URINARY INCONTINENCE

Imagine that you are Kay, the home care nurse in the Care Plan on pages 1184–1185 of your text. Complete the *assessment* phase of the critical thinking model by writing your answers in the appropriate boxes of the model shown. Think about the following:

- What knowledge base was applied to the care of Mrs. Grayson?
- In what ways might Kay's previous experience assist in this case?
- What intellectual or professional standards were applied to Mrs. Grayson?
- What critical thinking attitudes did you utilize in assessing Mrs. Grayson?
- As you review the assessment, what key areas did Kay cover?

Copyright © 2019 Elsevier Canada, a division of Reed Elsevier Canada, Ltd.

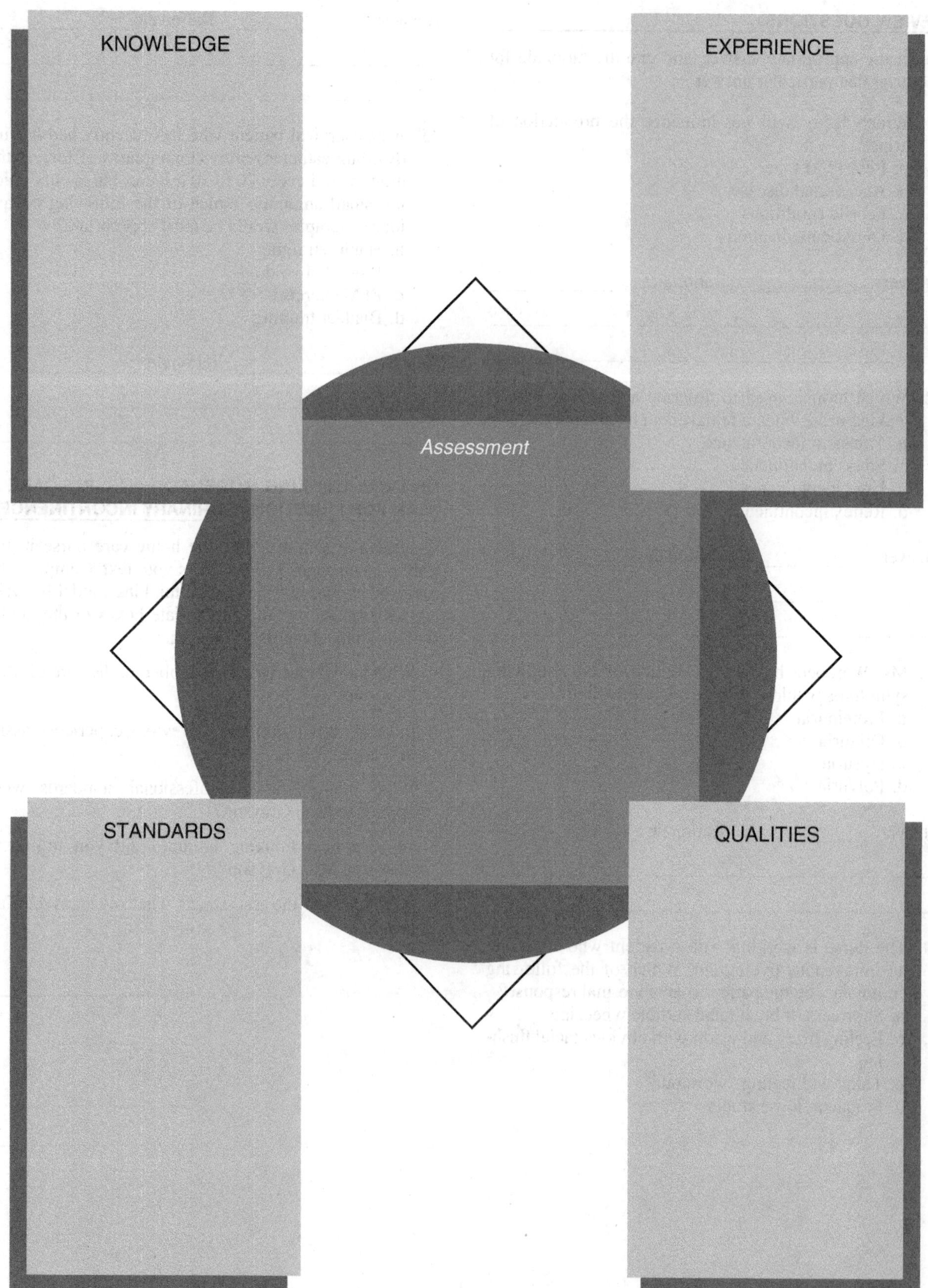

CHAPTER 43 Critical Thinking Model for Nursing Care Plan for *Functional Urinary Incontinence*
See answers on Evolve site.

Copyright © 2019 Elsevier Canada, a division of Reed Elsevier Canada, Ltd.

44 Bowel Elimination

PRELIMINARY READING

Chapter 44, pages 1211–1245

COMPREHENSIVE UNDERSTANDING

Scientific Knowledge Base

The gastrointestinal (GI) tract is a series of hollow, multilayered, muscular organs that are lined with mucous membranes.

1. Summarize the functions of the following organs.

   a. Mouth:

   b. Esophagus:

   c. Stomach:

   d. Small intestine:

   e. Large intestine:

2. Define the following terms and identify the portion of the GI tract to which they relate.

   a. *Masticate*:

   b. *Bolus*:

   c. *Peristalsis*:

   d. *Chyme*:

   e. *Flatus*:

   f. *Feces*:

Nursing Knowledge Base

Process of defecation

3. Indicate with numbers the correct sequence of mechanisms involved in normal defecation.

   _________ Abdominal muscles contract, increasing intrarectal pressure.

   _________ The external sphincter relaxes.

   _________ The internal sphincter relaxes, and awareness of the need to defecate occurs.

   _________ Movement in the left colon occurs, moving stool toward the anus.

4. Describe the *Valsalva manoeuvre* and the risk it poses to certain patients.

5. Describe how the squatting position facilitates defecation.

Copyright © 2019 Elsevier Canada, a division of Reed Elsevier Canada, Ltd.

Promotion of normal defecation

Several interventions can stimulate the defecation reflex, affect the character of feces, or increase peristalsis to help patients evacuate bowel contents normally and without discomfort.

6. List three interventions to facilitate defecation when using a bedpan.

   a. ______________________

   b. ______________________

   c. ______________________

7. Explain how the following can assist the patient to evacuate his or her bowels.

   a. Sitting position:

   ____

   b. Positioning on the bedpan:

   ____

8. Explain the proper technique for positioning a patient on a bedpan.

   ____

Factors affecting normal bowel elimination

Diet

9. Identify the mechanisms that cause high-fibre diets to promote elimination.

   ____

10. List three types of foods that are considered high in fibre (bulk).

    a. ______________________

    b. ______________________

    c. ______________________

11. Define *lactose intolerance.*

    ____

Fluid Intake

12. Summarize how an inadequate intake of fluids can affect the character of feces.

    ____

Physical Activity

13. Physical activity ______________ peristalsis; immobilization ______________ peristalsis.

14. Weakened abdominal and pelvic floor muscles impair the ability to ______________ and to ______________.

Personal Bowel Elimination Habits

15. List four personal elimination habits that influence bowel function.

    a. ______________________

    b. ______________________

    c. ______________________

    d. ______________________

Privacy

The patient's privacy must be maintained during bowel elimination.

Nursing Process and Bowel Elimination

Assessment

Health history

What a patient defines as "normal" may differ from factors and conditions that typically promote normal bowel elimination. You can determine the patient's problems by first identifying the normal and abnormal patterns and habits, and then understanding the patient's perception of normal and abnormal regarding bowel elimination.

16. List 16 factors affecting elimination that need to be included in a health history for patients with altered elimination status.

    a. ______________________

    b. ______________________

    c. ______________________

    d. ______________________

    e. ______________________

    f. ______________________

    g. ______________________

    h. ______________________

Copyright © 2019 Elsevier Canada, a division of Reed Elsevier Canada, Ltd.

i. ____________________

j. ____________________

k. ____________________

l. ____________________

m. ____________________

n. ____________________

o. ____________________

p. ____________________

Physical assessment

17. Summarize the following steps for assessing the abdomen.

a. Inspection:

____

____

b. Percussion:

____

____

c. Auscultation:

____

____

d. Palpation:

____

____

18. Summarize the assessment of the rectum.

____

____

____

____

Factors related to altered patterns of bowel elimination

Age-Related Changes

19. List five changes that occur in the GI system of the older persons that impair normal digestion and elimination.

a. ____________________

b. ____________________

c. ____________________

d. ____________________

e. ____________________

Infectious Disease

20. Microbial agents, including viruses, bacteria, and protozoa, can infect the GI tract. These infections can cause diarrhea and inflammatory or ulcerative changes in the small or large intestine. Most infections are spread by the __________ through __________ or __________.

21. List four infection control procedures to be taken with the *Norwalk virus*.

a. ____________________

b. ____________________

c. ____________________

d. ____________________

Irritable Bowel Syndrome

22. Management of irritable bowel syndrome is __________, based on the patient's most troublesome symptoms.

Diabetes

23. Patients with diabetes frequently report problems with constipation and/or diarrhea due to __________.

Pain

24. List conditions that may result in painful defecation.

a. ____________________

b. ____________________

c. ____________________

d. ____________________

Pelvic Floor Trauma

25. Identify the common problems related to defecation that occur during pregnancy, and explain why they occur.

____

____

____

____

____

Acute Illness, Surgery, and Anaesthesia

26. Summarize the effects of anaesthetic agents and peristalsis on defecation.

____

____

____

____

Copyright © 2019 Elsevier Canada, a division of Reed Elsevier Canada, Ltd.

Enteral Feeding

27. Discuss the etiology of diarrhea and constipation in patients receiving their nutrition through enteral feedings.

Medications That Affect Elimination

28. Describe the effect on elimination of each of the following medications.

    a. Opioids:

    b. Anticholinergics:

    c. Antibiotics:

    d. Nonsteroidal anti inflammatory drugs:

    e. Histamines:

    f. Proton pump inhibitor:

    g. Iron:

    h. Calcium carbonate:

Laboratory tests

Fecal Specimens

29. Briefly describe the appropriate technique for collecting a fecal specimen.

30. Define *fecal occult blood test.*

Fecal Characteristics

31. Describe the normal fecal characteristics.

    a. Colour:

    b. Odour:

    c. Consistency:

    d. Frequency:

    e. Shape:

    f. Constituents:

32. Indicate the possible cause for each of the following abnormal fecal characteristics.

    a. White or clay colour:

    b. Black and tarry (melena):

    c. Liquid consistency:

    d. Narrow, pencil-shaped:

Copyright © 2019 Elsevier Canada, a division of Reed Elsevier Canada, Ltd.

Diagnostic examinations

Diagnostic Tests

33. List three types of diagnostic tests for visualization of GI structures.
    a. ____
    b. ____
    c. ____

Nursing Diagnosis

34. List five potential or actual nursing diagnoses for a patient with alterations in bowel elimination.
    a. ____
    b. ____
    c. ____
    d. ____
    e. ____

Common bowel elimination problems

35. List five factors that place a patient at risk for elimination problems.
    a. ____
    b. ____
    c. ____
    d. ____
    e. ____

Constipation

36. Define *constipation.*

____

37. List and briefly describe four causes of constipation.
    a. ____
    b. ____
    c. ____
    d. ____

38. List three groups of patients in whom constipation could pose a significant health hazard.
    a. ____
    b. ____
    c. ____

Impaction

39. Define *fecal impaction.*

____

40. List four signs and symptoms of fecal impaction.
    a. ____
    b. ____
    c. ____
    d. ____

Diarrhea

41. Define *diarrhea.*

____

42. List four conditions that cause diarrhea.
    a. ____
    b. ____
    c. ____
    d. ____

43. Name the major complications associated with diarrhea.

____

Incontinence

44. Define *bowel incontinence.*

____

Flatulence

45. Flatulence results from ____. It is a common cause of ____, ____, and ____.

Hemorrhoids

46. Define *hemorrhoids.*

____

Copyright © 2019 Elsevier Canada, a division of Reed Elsevier Canada, Ltd.

47. List four conditions that cause hemorrhoids.

a. ____

b. ____

c. ____

d. ____

Planning

Goals and outcomes

48. List an example of a goal and five associated outcomes appropriate for patients with elimination problems.

a. ____

b. ____

c. ____

d. ____

e. ____

Implementation

Defecation patterns vary among individuals. For this reason, you and your patient must work together closely to plan effective interventions.

Teach the patient and the patient's family about proper diet, adequate fluid intake, and factors that stimulate or slow peristalsis, such as emotional stress.

Patient expectations

Patients expect a knowledgeable nurse who can teach them methods of promoting and maintaining a normal bowel elimination pattern.

Management of bowel elimination

Maintenance of Proper Fluid and Food Intake

Daily fluid intake should be between 1500 and 2000 mL of noncaffeinated beverages. Dietary fibre intake should be from 25 to 30 g/day.

49. Identify four interventions to reduce the risk of constipation.

a. ____

b. ____

c. ____

d. ____

Promotion of Regular Exercise

Walking, riding a stationary bicycle, or swimming stimulates peristalsis. Patients who are sedentary at work are most in need of regular exercise.

Bowel Retraining

50. Briefly explain *bowel retraining.*

____

____

____

____

51. Describe two nursing interventions that promote comfort for patients who experience the following:

a. Hemorrhoids:

____

____

b. Risks to skin integrity:

____

____

Medications

52. Identify the primary action of the following medications.

a. Cathartics:

____

____

b. Laxatives:

____

____

c. Antidiarrheals:

____

____

Enemas

53. The primary reason for an enema is

____.

54. Briefly describe the following types of enemas.

a. Tap water:

____

____

____

b. Normal saline:

____

____

____

c. Hypertonic solution:

____

____

____

Copyright © 2019 Elsevier Canada, a division of Reed Elsevier Canada, Ltd.

d. Soapsuds:

e. Oil retention:

f. Carminative:

Enema Administration

55. Explain the physician's order "Give enemas until clear."

56. List four complications of digital removal of stool.

a.
b.
c.
d.

Surgical management of bowel elimination

57. List four reasons to insert a nasogastric tube for decompression.

a.
b.
c.
d.

58. Explain how the Salem sump tube works.

Bowel diversions

59. Define the following terms.

a. *Stoma*:

b. *Ileostomy*:

c. *Colostomy*:

The location of the ostomy determines the consistency of the stool.

60. Briefly explain each of the following types of colostomy construction.

a. Loop colostomy:

b. End colostomy:

c. Double-barrel colostomy:

61. Briefly describe the *Kock continent ileostomy*.

Psychologic Considerations

62. Identify a major psychologic concern of a patient with an ostomy.

Care of Ostomies

63. Define *effluent*.

Copyright © 2019 Elsevier Canada, a division of Reed Elsevier Canada, Ltd.

Pouching Ostomies

64. List nine factors to consider when selecting a pouching system for a patient.

a. ______
b. ______
c. ______
d. ______
e. ______
f. ______
g. ______
h. ______
i. ______

Nutritional Considerations for Patients With Ostomies

65. Summarize the nutritional considerations for patients with ostomies.

______

Evaluation

Patient care

The effectiveness of care depends on success in meeting the goals and expected outcomes of care.

The patient is the only one who is able to determine if the bowel elimination problems have been relieved and which therapies were the most effective.

Patient expectations

The patient will relate a feeling of comfort and freedom from pain as elimination needs are met within the limits of the patient's condition and treatment.

REVIEW QUESTIONS

Select the appropriate answer, and cite the rationale for choosing that particular answer.

1. Which term best describes the slow-mixing contractions that move contents and expose chyme to mucosa?
   a. Flatus
   b. Peristalsis
   c. Emulsification
   d. Mastication

Answer: ______ Rationale: ______

2. Which of the following does *not* describe diagnostic examinations that involve visualization of the lower GI structures?
   a. The patient must drink fluids immediately before the test.
   b. The patient will probably receive a prescribed bowel preparation before the test.
   c. The patient is not allowed to eat or drink before the test.
   d. Changes in elimination may occur following the procedure until normal eating patterns resume.

Answer: ______ Rationale: ______

3. What would your first action be when caring for Mrs. Ahmed, who has secretory diarrhea?
   a. Administer Imodium
   b. Increase fluid intake with clear fluids
   c. Increase fluid intake with Gastrolyte
   d. Administer opiates, if prescribed

Answer: ______ Rationale: ______

4. What should you do next for your patient after positioning him or her on the bedpan?
   a. Leave the head of the bed flat
   b. Raise the head of the bed 30 degrees
   c. Raise the head of the bed to a 90-degree angle
   d. Raise the bed to the highest working level

Answer: ______ Rationale: ______

5. Which type of enema should the nurse administer if a cleansing enema has been ordered for 7-year-old Michael?
   a. Tap water enema
   b. Low-volume hypertonic saline enema
   c. Normal saline enema
   d. Soapsuds solution enema

Answer: ______ Rationale: ______

Copyright © 2019 Elsevier Canada, a division of Reed Elsevier Canada, Ltd.

CRITICAL THINKING MODEL FOR NURSING CARE PLAN FOR CONSTIPATION

Imagine that you are Javier, the home care nurse in the Care Plan on page 1228 of your text. Complete the *planning* phase of the critical thinking model by writing your answers in the appropriate boxes of the model shown. Think about the following:

- In developing Larry's plan of care, what knowledge did Javier apply?
- In what way might Javier's previous experience assist in developing a plan of care for Larry?
- When developing a plan of care, what intellectual or professional standards were applied?
- What critical thinking attitudes might have been applied in developing a plan for Larry?
- How will Javier accomplish the goals?

Copyright © 2019 Elsevier Canada, a division of Reed Elsevier Canada, Ltd.

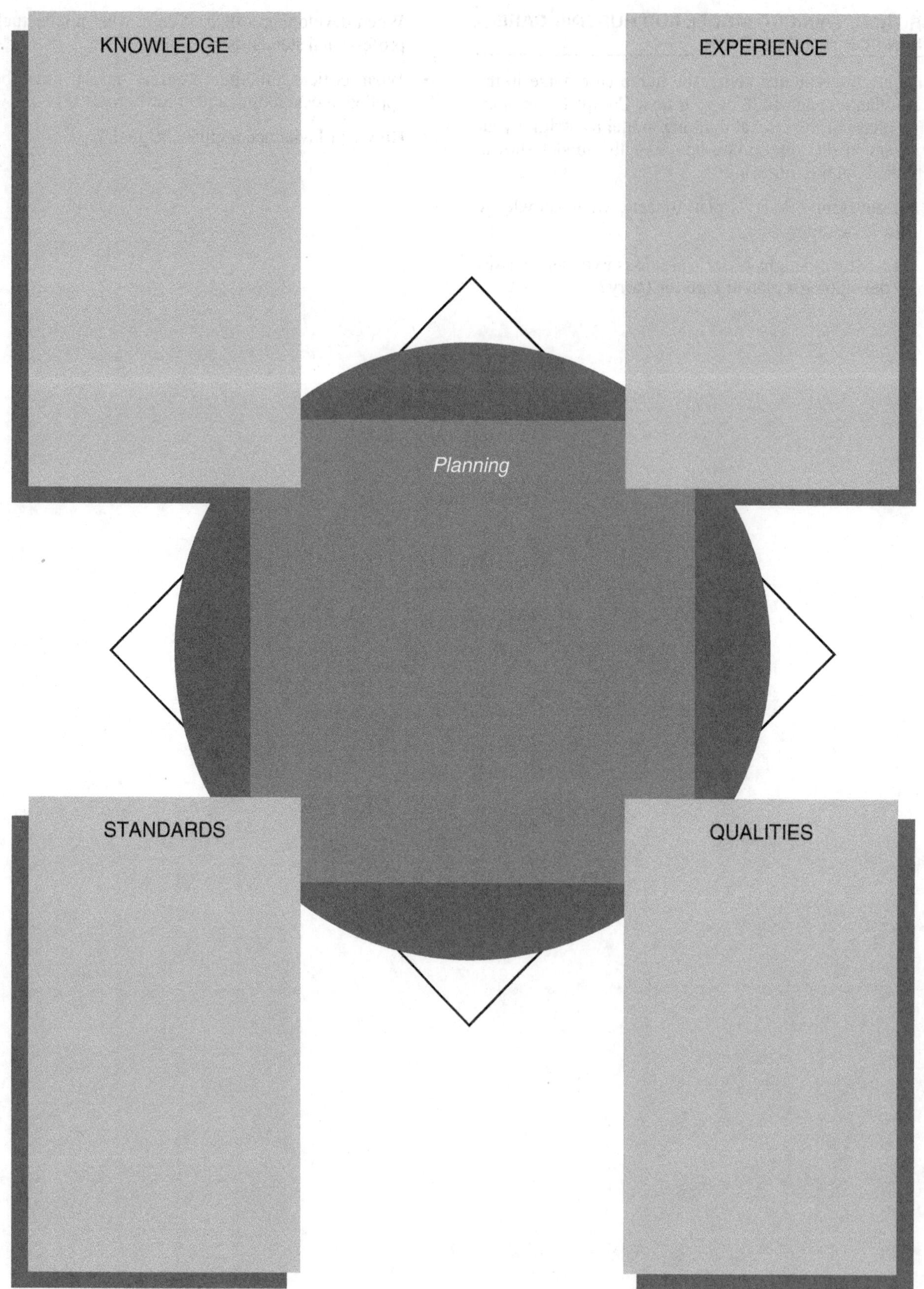

CHAPTER 44 Critical Thinking Model for Nursing Care Plan for *Constipation*
See answers on Evolve site.

Copyright © 2019 Elsevier Canada, a division of Reed Elsevier Canada, Ltd.

45 Mobility and Immobility

PRELIMINARY READING

Chapter 45, pages 1246–1287

COMPREHENSIVE UNDERSTANDING

1. *Mobility* refers to ______________________.

Scientific Knowledge Base

Physiology and principles of body mechanics

2. Define the following terms.
   a. *Body mechanics*: ______________________
   b. *Body alignment or posture*: ______________________
3. Balance is required for ______________________ ______, and for ______________________.
4. What compromises the ability to remain balanced? ______________________

Gravity and Friction

5. Define *friction*. ______________________
6. List two techniques that minimize friction.
   a. ______________________
   b. ______________________

Pathologic influences on mobility

7. Briefly explain how the following pathologic conditions affect mobility.
   a. Postural abnormalities: ______________________
   b. Impaired muscle development: ______________________
   c. Damage to the central nervous system: ______________________
   d. Direct trauma to the musculoskeletal system: ______________________
8. Describe *pathologic fractures.* ______________________

Nursing Knowledge Base

Mobility–immobility

9. *Mobility* refers to ______________________, and *immobility* refers to ______________________.
10. Define *bed rest.* ______________________

Copyright © 2019 Elsevier Canada, a division of Reed Elsevier Canada, Ltd.

11. *Impaired physical mobility* is defined as ____.

Developmental Changes

12. Identify the descriptive characteristics of body alignment and mobility related to the following developmental stages.

    a. Infants, toddlers, and preschoolers:

    b. Adolescents:

    c. Adults:

    d. Older persons:

13. Briefly describe the areas of functional decline in hospitalized older persons.

    a. Musculoskeletal:

    b. Elimination:

    c. Nutrition:

    d. Psychosocial:

Nursing Process for Impaired Body Alignment and Mobility

Assessment

14. Briefly describe the four major areas for assessment of patient mobility.

    a. Range of motion:

    b. Gait:

    c. Exercise and activity tolerance:

    d. Body alignment:

Immobility

Physiologic Assessment

15. Briefly describe the physiologic hazards of immobility in relation to the following systems.

    a. Metabolic:

    b. Respiratory:

    c. Cardiovascular:

    d. Musculoskeletal:

    e. Elimination:

    f. Integumentary:

Nursing Diagnosis

16. List six actual or potential nursing diagnoses related to an immobilized or partially immobilized patient.

    a. ____________________

    b. ____________________

    c. ____________________

    d. ____________________

    e. ____________________

    f. ____________________

Copyright © 2019 Elsevier Canada, a division of Reed Elsevier Canada, Ltd.

Planning

Goals and outcomes

The goals and expected outcomes are developed to assist the patient in achieving his or her highest level of mobility.

Setting priorities

17. The nurse plans therapies according to the severity of risks to the patient, and the plan is individualized according to the patient's ______________________, ______________, and ______________________.

Implementation

Health promotion

18. Briefly explain the benefits of *exercise*.

Acute care

19. Identify two nursing interventions to meet each of the following goals for the immobilized patient.
    a. Maintain optimal nutritional (metabolic) state:
    b. Promote expansion of the chest and lungs:
    c. Prevent stasis of pulmonary secretions:
    d. Maintain a patent airway:
    e. Reduce orthostatic hypotension:
    f. Reduce cardiac workload:
    g. Prevent thrombus formation:
    h. Maintain muscle strength and joint mobility:
    i. Maintain normal elimination patterns:
    j. Prevent pressure ulcers:
    k. Maintain usual psychosocial state:

20. Identify two nursing interventions for the immobilized child.
    a. ______________________
    b. ______________________

Positioning Devices and Techniques

21. Describe the following positions.
    a. Supported Fowlers:
    b. Supine:
    c. Prone:
    d. Side-lying:
    e. Sims:

Transfer Techniques

22. List some general guidelines to apply in any transfer procedure.

Copyright © 2019 Elsevier Canada, a division of Reed Elsevier Canada, Ltd.

Repositioning Patients

Always enlist the patient's help to the fullest extent possible.

23. List four areas the nurse needs to consider in determining if assistance is required when repositioning a patient in bed.
    a. ______
    b. ______
    c. ______
    d. ______

Transferring a Patient from a Bed to a Stretcher

To transfer a patient who is immobile from a bed to a stretcher or from a bed to another bed, use a friction-reducing device under the patient.

Restorative Care

24. The goal of restorative care for the immobile patient is to ______ ______.

25. Instrumental activities of daily living are ______ ______.

Joint Mobility

Range-of-Motion Exercises

26. Indicate the type of joint and range-of-motion exercises for the body parts listed in the following table.

Body Part	Type of Joint	Type of Movement
Neck		
Shoulder		
Forearm		
Wrist		
Fingers and thumb		
Hip		
Knee		
Ankle and foot		
Toes		

Copyright © 2019 Elsevier Canada, a division of Reed Elsevier Canada, Ltd.

Evaluation

Patient care

To evaluate outcomes, the nurse measures the effectiveness of all interventions. The actual outcomes are compared with the outcomes selected during planning.

The optimal outcomes are the patient's ability to maintain or improve body alignment and joint mobility.

Patient expectations

Patient expectations evaluate care from the patient's perspective.

REVIEW QUESTIONS

Select the appropriate answer, and cite the rationale for choosing that particular answer.

1. Which of the following physiologic effects of exercise on the body systems would the nurse *not* expect?
   a. Decreased cardiac output
   b. Increased respiratory rate and depth
   c. Increased muscle tone, size, and strength
   d. Change in metabolic rate

Answer:______________ Rationale:______________

____

____

2. Which of the following is a potential hazard for which the nurse should assess when the patient is in the prone position?
   a. Unprotected pressure points at the sacrum and heels
   b. Internal rotation of the shoulder
   c. Increased cervical flexion
   d. Plantar flexion

Answer:______________ Rationale:______________

____

____

3. Which of the following is a physiologic effect of prolonged bed rest?
   a. A decrease in urinary excretion of nitrogen
   b. An increase in cardiac output
   c. A decrease in lean body mass
   d. A decrease in lung expansion

Answer:______________ Rationale:______________

____

____

4. Which of the following is *not* used to assess for deep-vein thrombosis?
   a. Measuring the circumference of each leg daily, placing the tape measure at the midpoint of the knee
   b. Observing the dorsal aspect of lower extremities for redness, warmth, and tenderness
   c. Asking the patient about the presence of calf pain
   d. Checking for a positive Homans sign, if not contraindicated

Answer:______________ Rationale:______________

____

____

5. Which group of interventions is aimed at the prevention of pressure ulcers?
   a. Teach patients to shift their weight in a chair every 2 hours.
   b. Reposition frequently and use therapeutic devices to relieve pressure.
   c. Turn patient every 15 minutes in bed and use a doughnut device.
   d. Rub skin vigorously to increase circulation and turn patient every 2 hours.

Answer:______________ Rationale:______________

____

____

6. Which of the following is an appropriate intervention to maintain the respiratory system of the immobilized patient?
   a. Turn the patient every 4 hours.
   b. Maintain a maximum fluid intake of 1500 mL per day.
   c. Apply and maintain an abdominal binder.
   d. Encourage the use of an incentive spirometer.

Answer:______________ Rationale:______________

____

____

CRITICAL THINKING MODEL FOR NURSING CARE PLAN FOR IMPAIRED PHYSICAL MOBILITY

Imagine that you are the student nurse in the Care Plan on pages 1265–1266 of your text. Complete the *evaluation* phase of the critical thinking model by writing your answers in the appropriate boxes of the model shown. Think about the following:

- What knowledge did you apply in evaluating Ms. Adams's care?
- In what way might your previous experience influence your evaluation of Ms. Adams?
- During evaluation, what intellectual and professional standards were applied to Ms. Adams's care?
- In what ways do critical thinking attitudes play a role in how you approach evaluation of Ms. Adams's care?
- How might you adjust Ms. Adams's care?

Copyright © 2019 Elsevier Canada, a division of Reed Elsevier Canada, Ltd.

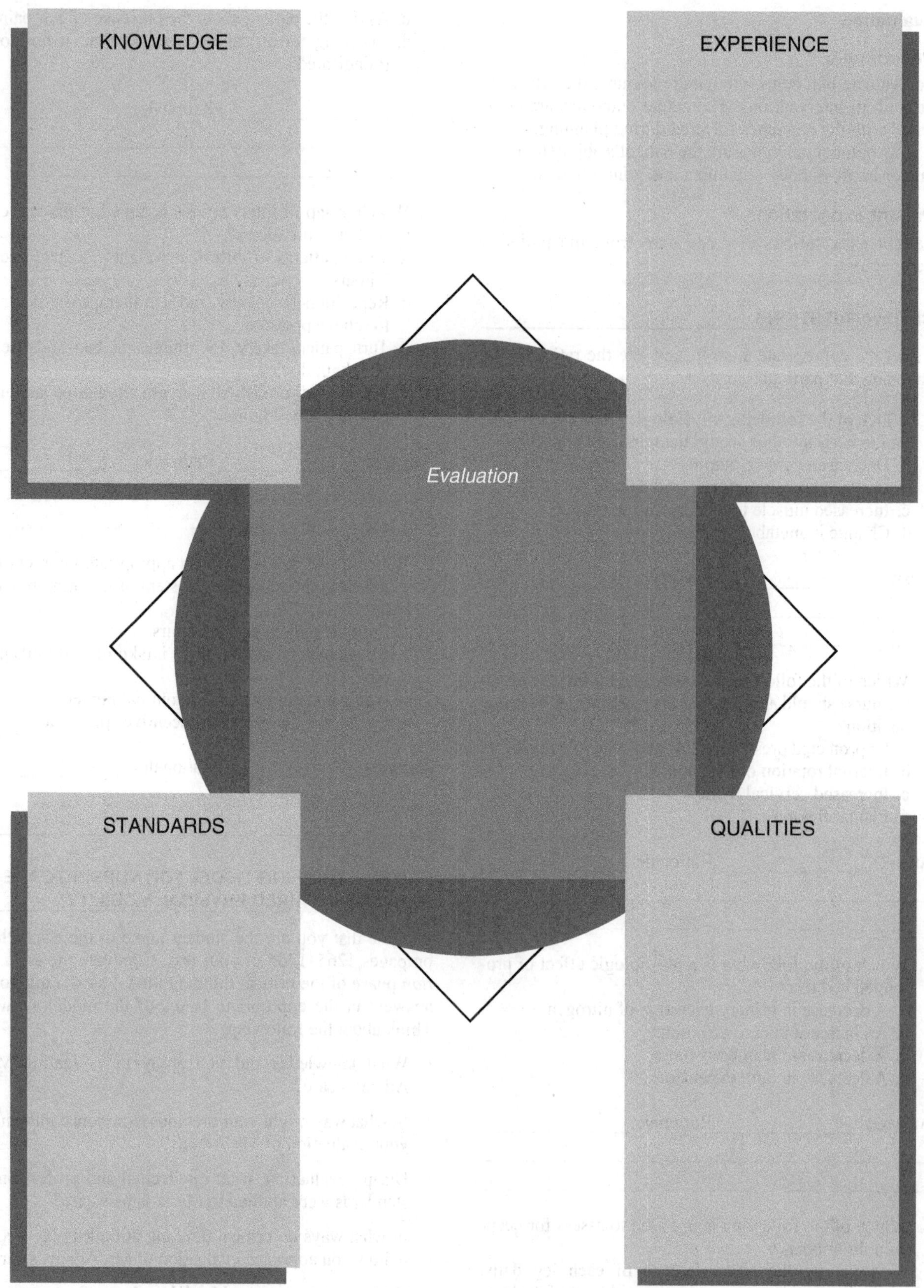

CHAPTER 45 Critical Thinking Model for Nursing Care Plan for *Impaired Physical Mobility*
See answers on Evolve site.

Copyright © 2019 Elsevier Canada, a division of Reed Elsevier Canada, Ltd.

46 Skin Integrity and Wound Care

PRELIMINARY READING

Chapter 46, pages 1288–1338

COMPREHENSIVE UNDERSTANDING

Scientific Knowledge Base

Skin

1. Describe the function of each of the following layers of skin.

   a. Epidermis:

   b. Dermis:

Pressure injury

2. Define *pressure injury*.

Pathogenesis of Pressure Ulcers

3. Identify the pressure factors that contribute to pressure injury development.

   a.

   b.

   c.

4. Define the following terms.

   a. *Hyperemia* (erythema):

   b. *Blanching*:

5. Explain the difference between normal reactive hyperemia and abnormal reactive hyperemia. Indicate which of the two is a sign of deep tissue damage.

Nursing Knowledge Base

Prediction and prevention of pressure injury

Consistent, planned skin care interventions are critical to ensuring high-quality care. You need to take every opportunity to observe and assess your patients' skin for impaired skin integrity.

Risk Factors for Pressure Injury Development

6. Briefly explain how the following factors contribute to an increased risk for pressure injury.

   a. Impaired sensory perception:

   b. Impaired mobility:

   c. Alteration in level of consciousness:

   d. Shear:

   e. Friction:

Copyright © 2019 Elsevier Canada, a division of Reed Elsevier Canada, Ltd.

f. Moisture:

g. Nutrition:

h. Tissue perfusion:

i. Infection:

j. Pain:

k. Age:

Psychosocial Impact of Wounds

7. Identify the factors that may affect the patient's perception of the wound.

Nursing Process

Assessment

Skin integrity is subject to change over time. Baseline and continual assessment data support critical information about the patient's skin integrity and the increased risk of pressure ulcer development.

Skin

8. What factors should be considered in each of the four areas when assessing skin integrity.

a. Sensation:

b. Mobility:

c. Continence:

d. Presence of a wound:

Risk assessment

Evidence exists that a program of prevention guided by consistent risk assessment simultaneously reduces the institutional incidence of pressure ulcers by as much as 60%.

Braden scale

9. List the six categories of the Braden scale used to predict for pressure ulcer risk.

a.

b.

c.

d.

e.

f.

Classification of pressure injury

10. A pressure injury is classified in stages according to its severity. Briefly describe the staging system devised by the National Pressure Ulcer Advisory Panel.

a. Suspected deep tissue injury:

b. Stage I:

c. Stage II:

Copyright © 2019 Elsevier Canada, a division of Reed Elsevier Canada, Ltd.

d. Stage III:

e. Stage IV:

f. Unstageable:

Wound classification

It is imperative that you understand that *all wounds are not created equal.* Understanding the etiology of a wound is important because the treatment for the wound varies depending on the underlying disease process. Some treatments are even harmful to certain wounds, so you always need to obtain a complete history, including the etiology of the wound.

Process of wound healing

11. Describe the physiologic process involved with wound healing.

a. Primary intention:

b. Secondary intention:

c. Tertiary intention:

Wound repair

Partial-Thickness Wound Repair

12. Explain the three components involved in the healing of a partial-thickness wound.

a.

b.

c.

Full-Thickness Wound Repair

13. Explain the three phases involved in the healing of a full-thickness wound.

a. Inflammatory phase:

b. Proliferative phase:

c. Remodelling:

14. Briefly describe the etiology of and two main treatment points to consider for each type of wound listed.

a. Skin tear:

b. Venous ulcer:

c. Arterial ulcer:

d. Diabetic ulcer:

e. Malignant or fungating wound:

f. Acute or surgical wound:

Copyright © 2019 Elsevier Canada, a division of Reed Elsevier Canada, Ltd.

Character of Wound Drainage

15. Describe the four major types of wound drainage (*exudate*).

    a. ______________________

    b. ______________________

    c. ______________________

    d. ______________________

Wound Cultures

16. What is the purpose of obtaining a wound culture?

    ____

17. Describe the method of obtaining a wound culture.

    ____

Complications of wound healing

18. Briefly explain the following complications of wound healing.

    a. Hemorrhage:

    b. Infection:

    c. Dehiscence:

    d. Evisceration:

    e. Fistulas:

19. What are the characteristics of wound infection?

    a. ______________________

    b. ______________________

    c. ______________________

    d. ______________________

    e. ______________________

Nursing Diagnosis

20. List three nursing diagnoses related to impaired skin integrity.

    a. ______________________

    b. ______________________

    c. ______________________

Planning

21. List six possible goals for the patient at risk for pressure ulcers.

    a. ______________________

    b. ______________________

    c. ______________________

    d. ______________________

    e. ______________________

    f. ______________________

Collaborative care

22. Discuss the information that should be provided when a patient is discharged or moves to another care setting.

    ____

Implementation: Preventing Skin Breakdown

23. Briefly explain the following nursing interventions for the prevention of pressure ulcers.

    a. Topical skin care:

    b. Positioning:

Copyright © 2019 Elsevier Canada, a division of Reed Elsevier Canada, Ltd.

c. Support surfaces (therapeutic beds and mattresses):

d. Education:

e. Management of pressure injury:

Wound management

Prevention of wound infection includes wound cleansing and removal of nonviable tissue (*debridement*).

24. List and explain the principles to follow when cleansing a wound or the area around a drain.

25. ______ is a common method of delivering the wound cleansing solution to the wound.

Studies have shown that an optimal effective range of irrigation pressures exists that ensures adequate removal of bacteria. To ensure an irrigation pressure within the correct range, use a 35-mL syringe with a 19-gauge angiocatheter or a single 100-mL saline squeeze bottle.

26. Describe the following methods of debridement.

a. Mechanical:

b. Biologic:

c. Chemical or enzymatic:

d. Autolytic:

e. Surgical:

Nutritional Status

27. List four recommendations for nutritional assessment and management of pressure injury in the malnourished patient.

a.

b.

c.

d.

Protein Status

28. Patients require a higher intake of the following to promote healing.

a.

b.

c.

Dressings

29. List the purposes for dressings.

a.

b.

c.

d.

e.

f.

g.

30. List the clinical guidelines to use when selecting the appropriate dressing.

a.

b.

c.

d.

e.

f.

31. Briefly describe the following types of dressings and their uses.

a. Woven gauze:

b. Transparent film:

Copyright © 2019 Elsevier Canada, a division of Reed Elsevier Canada, Ltd.

c. Nonadherent contact layer:

____

____

d. Soft silicone:

____

____

e. Hydrocolloid:

____

____

f. Hydrogel:

____

____

g. Foam:

____

____

h. Calcium alginate:

____

____

i. Composite:

____

____

j. Topical treatment:

____

____

k. Hypertonic:

____

____

l. Cadexomer iodine:

____

____

m. Silver:

____

____

n. Honey:

____

____

o. Gentian violet/methylene blue:

____

____

p. Negative-pressure wound therapy:

____

____

32. To prepare for a dressing change, you should be familiar with the ______________________________

______________________________, and ______________

______________________________.

Clean or Sterile Technique

The RNAO guidelines (2011) recommend sterile dressings, good handwashing, and clean gloves changed between each of the patient's wounds or when soiled.

33. List the activities you would perform to prepare a patient for a dressing change.
    a. ______________________________
    b. ______________________________
    c. ______________________________
    d. ______________________________
    e. ______________________________

Packing a Wound

34. The first step in packing a wound is to assess the ______________, ______________, and ______________ of the wound.

35. Summarize the principles of packing a wound.

____

____

____

____

____

____

Securing Dressings

36. A dressing may be secured by ______________, ______________, ______________, or ______________.

Surgical or traumatic wound considerations

37. Summarize the nursing responsibilities for *suture* care.

____

____

____

____

Copyright © 2019 Elsevier Canada, a division of Reed Elsevier Canada, Ltd.

38. The manner in which the suture ________ and ________ the skin determines the ________.

39. Discuss the suture removal procedure.

____

Drainage Evacuation

40. Explain the purpose for drainage evacuation.

____

Bandages and Binders

41. Explain how bandages and binders applied over or around dressings provide extra protection and therapeutic benefits.

a. ________
b. ________
c. ________
d. ________
e. ________
f. ________

Principles for Applying Bandages and Binders

42. List the nursing responsibilities when applying a bandage or binder.

a. ________
b. ________
c. ________
d. ________

Abdominal Binders

43. Describe the *abdominal binder*.

____

Evaluation

You evaluate nursing interventions for reducing and treating pressure injury by determining the patient's response to nursing therapies and whether the patient achieved each goal.

44. The optimal outcomes are to ________, ________, and ________.

REVIEW QUESTIONS

Select the appropriate answer, and cite the rationale for choosing that particular answer.

1. Which of the following best defines ischemia?
   a. Increased tissue buildup during the healing process
   b. A reduction of blood flow to the tissues
   c. Decreased fluid to the tissues
   d. Increased irritability of nerves

Answer: ________ Rationale: ________

2. Mr. Prada is in a Fowler position to improve his oxygenation status. You note that he frequently slides down in the bed and needs to be repositioned. What is contributing to Mr. Prada's risk for developing a pressure ulcer on his coccyx?
   a. Friction
   b. Shearing force
   c. Maceration
   d. Impaired peripheral circulation

Answer: ________ Rationale: ________

3. Which of the following is *not* a subscale on the Braden Scale for predicting skin breakdown risk?
   a. Age
   b. Sensory perception
   c. Moisture
   d. Activity

Answer: ________ Rationale: ________

4. Which of the following patients has a nutritional risk for pressure injury development?
   a. Patient A has a serum albumin level of 37 g/L.
   b. Patient B has a lymphocyte count of $2000/mm^3$.
   c. Patient C has a body mass index of 17.
   d. Patient D has a body weight that is 5% greater than his ideal weight.

Answer: ________ Rationale: ________

Copyright © 2019 Elsevier Canada, a division of Reed Elsevier Canada, Ltd.

5. Mrs. Tootoosis is an immobilized patient. Which of the following will *not* increase her risk of developing a pressure ulcer?
   a. She has unrelieved pressure to her hip of greater than 32 mm Hg.
   b. After being turned to her side, she displays normal reactive hyperemia on her coccyx that lasts for 5 minutes.
   c. She has low-intensity pressure over a long period to her heels as a result of elastic stockings.
   d. She is positioned so that she has an unequal distribution of body weight.

Answer:______________ Rationale:______________

6. Mr. Wong has a stage II injury of his right heel. What would be the most appropriate treatment for this injury?
   a. Apply a thick layer of enzymatic ointment to the ulcer and the surrounding skin.
   b. Apply a calcium alginate dressing, and change when strikethrough is noted.
   c. Apply a heat lamp to the area for 20 minutes twice daily.
   d. Apply a hydrocolloid dressing and change it as necessary.

Answer:______________ Rationale:______________

Copyright © 2019 Elsevier Canada, a division of Reed Elsevier Canada, Ltd.

47 Sensory Alterations

PRELIMINARY READING

Chapter 47, pages 1339–1362

COMPREHENSIVE UNDERSTANDING

1. Define *stereognosis.*

Scientific Knowledge Base

Normal sensation

2. List and briefly explain the three functional components necessary for any sensory experience.
   a.
   b.
   c.

Sensory alterations

3. The types of sensory alterations commonly seen by the nurse are ________, ________, and ________.

Sensory Deficits

4. Define *sensory deficit.*

5. For each of the following, describe a disease or condition that may cause it.
   a. Visual deficit:
   b. Hearing deficit:
   c. Balance deficit:
   d. Taste deficit:

Sensory deprivation

6. List the three major types of sensory deprivation and give an example of each.
   a.
   b.
   c.

Sensory Overload

7. Define *sensory overload.*

8. Identify the behavioural changes that are associated with sensory overload.

Copyright © 2019 Elsevier Canada, a division of Reed Elsevier Canada, Ltd.

Nursing Knowledge Base

Factors affecting sensory function

9. Explain how and why the following factors affect sensory function.

 a. Age:

 b. Stimuli (quantity and quality):

 c. Family support:

 d. Environment:

 e. Medications:

 f. Ethnicity:

Nursing Process

Assessment

10. The nurse collects a history that assesses the patient's current sensory status and the degree to which a sensory deficit affects the patient's ____________, ____________, ____________, ____________, and ____________.

Use of assistive devices

11. Explain the measures taken to ensure that assistive devices (e.g., hearing aids and glasses) being used help maintain sensory function at the highest level.

12. The most common visual problem is ____________.

13. List the three recommended vision screening interventions.

 a. ____________

 b. ____________

 c. ____________

14. Explain how hearing loss can be caused by exposure to excessive noise.

Mental status

15. When assessing the patient's mental status, you need to evaluate each of the following. Give an example of each.

 a. Physical appearance and behaviour:

 b. Cognitive ability:

 c. Emotional status:

Copyright © 2019 Elsevier Canada, a division of Reed Elsevier Canada, Ltd.

16. Complete the grid that follows by describing at least one assessment technique for the identified sensory function and the behaviours for an adult and child that would indicate a sensory deficit.

Sense	Assessment Technique	Child Behaviour	Adult Behaviour
Vision			
Hearing			
Touch			
Smell			
Taste			
Position sense			

Physical assessment

17. Give an example of an assessment for the following that might assist you in deciding if the patient has a sensory alteration.

a. Ability to perform self-care:

b. Health promotion habits:

c. Hazards:

Hazards

18. List some examples of the more common hazards for a patient with sensory alterations.

a.

b.

c.

d.

e.

f.

g.

h.

i.

j.

k.

Communication methods

To understand the nature of a communication problem, you must know whether a patient has trouble speaking, understanding, naming, reading, or writing. Patients with existing sensory deficits often develop alternative ways of communicating.

Nursing Diagnosis

19. List six or more actual or potential nursing diagnoses that might apply to a patient with sensory alterations.

a.

b.

c.

d.

e.

f.

g.

h.

Planning

Goals and outcomes

20. List an example of a goal and four associated outcomes appropriate for a patient with a sensory alteration.

Goal:

Outcomes:

a.

b.

c.

d.

e.

Copyright © 2019 Elsevier Canada, a division of Reed Elsevier Canada, Ltd.

Preventive Safety

21. Identify the common injuries due to trauma that result in hearing or vision loss in both adults and children.
    a. Adults:
    b. Children:

22. List methods of establishing a safe environment with regard to the following:
    a. Adaptations for visual loss:
    b. Adaptations for reduced hearing:
    c. Adaptations for reduced taste and olfaction:
    d. Adaptations for reduced tactile sensation:
    e. Adaptations to the environment:

Promoting Self-Care

23. Often family members and nurses believe that patients with sensory impairments require assistance when, in fact, they can help themselves. Provide some useful guidelines to assist patients so they can help themselves with daily living activities.
    a. Visual assistance:
    b. Tactile assistance:
    c. Proprioceptive:

Evaluation

Patient care

Only patients themselves will know if their sensory abilities are improved and which interventions or therapies are the most successful.

Patient expectations

24. Patient expectations are one of the evaluative criteria used by the nurse. What questions might you ask to determine if patient expectations have been met?

REVIEW QUESTIONS

Select the appropriate answer, and cite the rationale for choosing that particular answer.

1. Which one of the following is *not true* of age-related factors that influence sensory function?
   a. Refractive errors are the most common types of visual disorders in children.
   b. Visual changes in adulthood include presbyopia.
   c. Older persons hear high-pitched sounds best.
   d. Neonates are unable to discriminate sensory stimuli.

Answer: ______ Rationale: ______

2. Mr. McDonald, a 62-year-old farmer, has been hospitalized for 2 weeks for thrombophlebitis. He has no visitors, and the nurse notices that he appears bored, restless, and anxious. What type of alteration is occurring because of sensory deprivation?
   a. Affective
   b. Cognitive
   c. Perceptual
   d. Receptive

Answer: ______ Rationale: ______

Copyright © 2019 Elsevier Canada, a division of Reed Elsevier Canada, Ltd.

3. Which of the following would *not* provide meaningful stimuli for a patient?
   a. A clock or calendar with large numbers
   b. A television that is kept on all day at a low volume
   c. Family pictures and personal possessions
   d. Interesting magazines and books

Answer: ____________ Rationale: ______________

____

____

4. Patients with existing sensory loss must be protected from injury. What determines the safety precautions taken?
   a. The existing dangers in the environment
   b. The financial means to make needed safety changes
   c. The nature of the patient's actual or potential sensory loss
   d. The availability of a support system to enable the patient to exist in his or her present environment

Answer: ____________ Rationale: ______________

____

____

5. Mr. Johnson is an 84-year-old postoperative patient with a hearing impairment. Methods to assist communication would include all but one of the following:
   a. Speak quickly and shout.
   b. Face the patient, and stand or sit on the same level.
   c. Rephrase when you are not understood.
   d. Avoid speaking from another room or while walking away.

Answer: ____________ Rationale: ______________

____

____

CRITICAL THINKING MODEL FOR NURSING CARE PLAN FOR DISTURBED SENSORY PERCEPTION

Imagine that you are the community health nurse in the Care Plan on pages 1353–1354 of your text. Complete the *planning* phase of the critical thinking model by writing your answers in the appropriate boxes of the model shown. Think about the following:

- In developing Judy's plan of care, what knowledge did you apply?
- In what way might your previous experience assist in developing a plan of care?
- When developing a plan of care, what intellectual and professional standards were applied?
- What critical thinking attitudes might have been applied in Judy's plan of care?
- How will you accomplish the goals?

Copyright © 2019 Elsevier Canada, a division of Reed Elsevier Canada, Ltd.

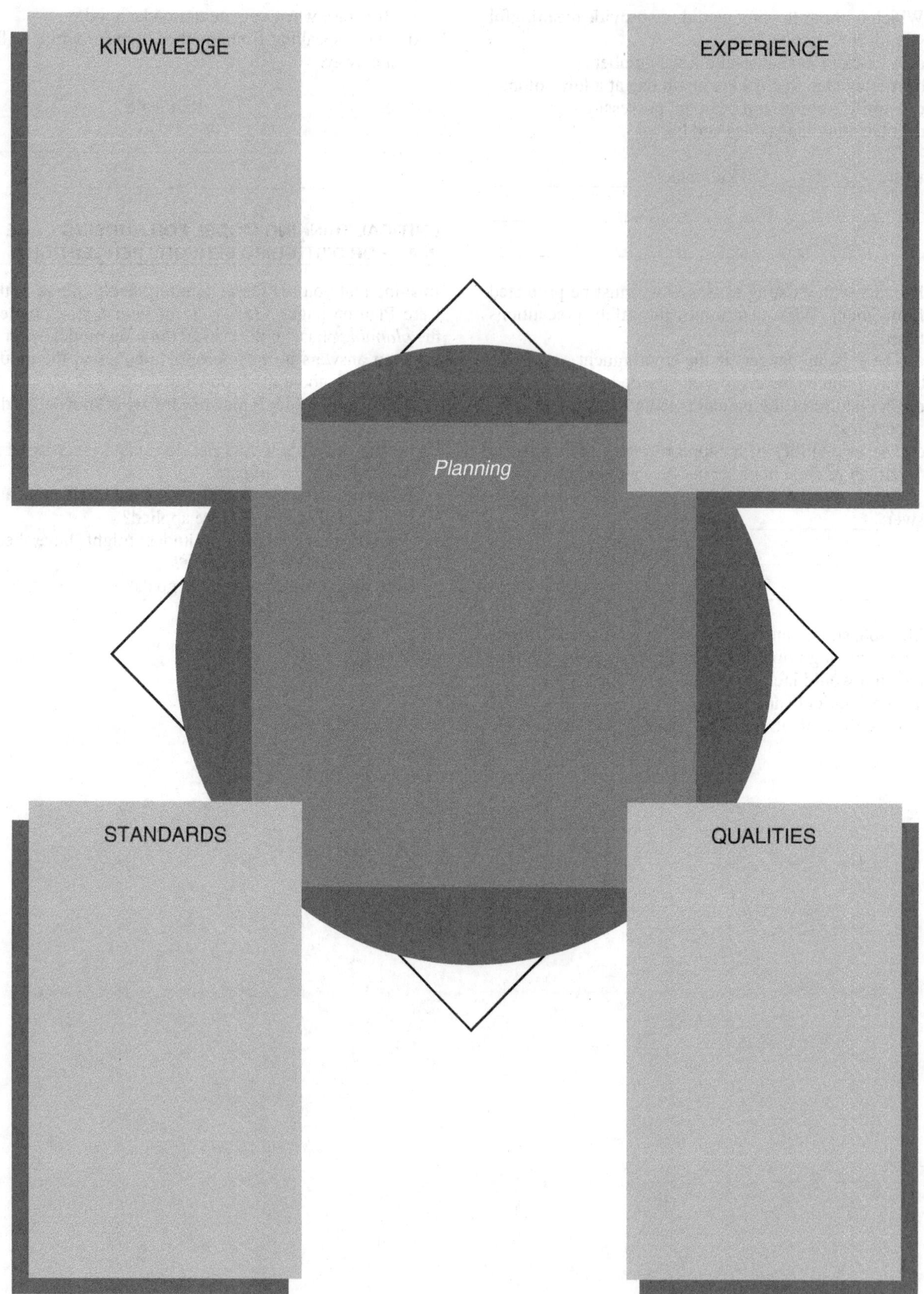

CHAPTER 47 Critical Thinking Model for Nursing Care Plan for *Disturbed Sensory Perception*
See answers on Evolve site.

Copyright © 2019 Elsevier Canada, a division of Reed Elsevier Canada, Ltd.

48 Care of Surgical Patients

PRELIMINARY READING

Chapter 48, pages 1363–1411

COMPREHENSIVE UNDERSTANDING

1. Define *perioperative nursing.*

History of Surgical Nursing

2. Summarize the historic changes that have occurred in surgical nursing.

Same-day (ambulatory) surgery

3. List the benefits of ambulatory surgery.
   a.
   b.
   c.
   d.

Scientific Knowledge Base

Classification of surgery

4. Define the following surgical procedure classifications.
   a. *Major surgery*:
   b. *Minor surgery*:
   c. *Elective surgery*:
   d. *Urgent surgery*:
   e. *Emergency surgery*:
   f. *Diagnostic surgery*:
   g. *Ablative surgery*:
   h. *Palliative surgery*:
   i. *Reconstructive or restorative surgery*:
   j. *Procurement for transplant*:
   k. *Constructive surgery*:
   l. *Cosmetic surgery*:

The Nursing Process in the Preoperative Surgical Phase

Assessment

An interprofessional team approach is essential. Patients are admitted only hours before the surgical event; thus you must organize and verify data obtained preoperatively to implement a perioperative care plan.

Medical history

5. Identify the data you should collect from the patient's medical history.

Copyright © 2019 Elsevier Canada, a division of Reed Elsevier Canada, Ltd.

Risk factors

6. Briefly explain the following factors that increase the patient's risk in surgery.

   a. Age:

   b. Nutrition:

   c. Obesity:

   d. Immunocompetence:

   e. Fluid and electrolyte imbalances:

   f. Pregnancy:

7. Briefly explain the rationale for assessing the following factors.

   a. Previous surgeries:

   b. Perceptions and understanding of surgery:

   c. Medication history:

   d. Allergies:

   e. Smoking habits:

   f. Alcohol ingestion and substance use and abuse:

   g. Family support:

   h. Occupation:

   i. Preoperative preparation for pain assessment and management:

Copyright © 2019 Elsevier Canada, a division of Reed Elsevier Canada, Ltd.

Review of emotional health

8. Briefly explain each of the following factors that must be assessed to understand the impact of surgery on a patient's and family's emotional health.

 a. Body image:

 b. Coping resources:

Culture

9. Cultural differences influence the surgical experience. Give an example.

Physical examination

10. Briefly describe the findings on which you should focus related to the physical examination of the following body systems.

 a. General survey:

 b. Head and neck:

 c. Integument:

 d. Thorax and lungs:

 e. Heart and vascular system:

 f. Abdomen:

 g. Neurologic status:

Diagnostic screening

11. Describe the following routine screening tests for surgical patients.

 a. Complete blood count:

 b. Serum electrolytes:

 c. Coagulation studies:

 d. Serum creatinine:

 e. Blood urea nitrogen:

 f. Glucose:

Nursing Diagnosis

12. List 10 potential or actual nursing diagnoses appropriate for the preoperative patient.

 a.

 b.

 c.

Copyright © 2019 Elsevier Canada, a division of Reed Elsevier Canada, Ltd.

d. ______
e. ______
f. ______
g. ______
h. ______
i. ______
j. ______

Planning

Goals and outcomes

13. Give examples of associated outcomes related to the goal of a preoperative patient being able to verbalize the significance of postoperative exercises.
   a. ______
   b. ______
   c. ______
   d. ______

Implementation

Informed consent

14. Surgery cannot be performed until a patient understands the following:
   a. ______
   b. ______
   c. ______
   d. ______
   e. ______

Preoperative teaching

Preparatory information helps patients anticipate the steps of a procedure and thus helps them form realistic images of the surgical experience. When events occur as predicted, patients are better able to cope and attend to the experiences.

15. Describe the criteria that may demonstrate the patient's understanding of the surgical procedure.
   a. ______
   b. ______
   c. ______
   d. ______
   e. ______
   f. ______
   g. ______
   h. ______

Acute care

Physical Preparation

16. Briefly describe the following preoperative preparations.
   a. Maintenance of normal fluid and electrolyte balances:
   ______
   b. Reduction of risk of surgical wound infection:
   ______
   c. Precautions for patient requiring infection-control procedures:
   ______
   d. Prevention of bowel incontinence:
   ______
   e. Promotion of rest and comfort:
   ______

Preparation on the Day of Surgery

17. List nine responsibilities of a nurse caring for a patient on the day of surgery.
   a. ______
   b. ______
   c. ______
   d. ______
   e. ______
   f. ______
   g. ______
   h. ______
   i. ______

Copyright © 2019 Elsevier Canada, a division of Reed Elsevier Canada, Ltd.

Latex Sensitivity or Allergy.

18. The signs and symptoms of a latex reaction are ______________________.

Eliminating Wrong Site and Wrong Procedure Surgery.

19. Describe methods to eliminate wrong site and wrong procedure surgery.

Transport to the Operating Room

20. After the patient leaves the nursing division, the nurse prepares the bed and room for the patient's return if the patient is returning to the same nursing division. List 10 pieces of equipment that should be present in the postoperative bedside unit.
    a. ______________________
    b. ______________________
    c. ______________________
    d. ______________________
    e. ______________________
    f. ______________________
    g. ______________________
    h. ______________________
    i. ______________________
    j. ______________________

Intraoperative Surgical Phase

21. The nurse functions in one of two roles in the OR: ______________ or ______________.

Preoperative (holding) area

22. In the holding area, two nursing responsibilities are ______________ and ______________ ______________________.

The Nursing Process in the Intraoperative Surgical Phase

Assessment

23. The preoperative assessment in the OR is important for the patient's safety because ______________________ ______________________.

Planning

Patient-centred outcomes of preoperative care extend into the intraoperative phase.

Implementation

Introduction of Anaesthesia

General Anaesthesia.

24. *General anaesthesia* involves ______________________.

Regional Anaesthesia.

25. *Regional anaesthesia* results in ______________________.

Local Anaesthesia.

26. *Local anaesthesia* involves ______________________.

Procedural Sedation.

27. Describe *procedural sedation,* and identify its advantages.

Positioning the Patient for Surgery

28. Identify factors to consider when positioning the patient for surgery.

Documentation of Intraoperative Care

During the intraoperative phase, the nursing staff continues the preoperative plan.

Documentation of intraoperative care provides useful data for the nurse who cares for the patient postoperatively.

Postoperative Surgical Phase

Immediate postoperative recovery

29. Describe the assessment data that you should obtain in the postanaesthesia care unit (PACU).

Copyright © 2019 Elsevier Canada, a division of Reed Elsevier Canada, Ltd.

Discharge from the PACU

30. Identify the criteria for discharge from the PACU.

a.
b.
c.
d.
e.
f.
g.
h.

Recovery in ambulatory surgery

31. Describe the two phases of postanaesthesia recovery.

a. Phase I:

b. Phase II:

32. Describe what the *Postanesthesia Recovery Score* tool is and what minimum score is required for discharge.

The Nursing Process in Postoperative Care

Assessment

33. Explain the frequency of assessments needed during the postoperative period.

Respiration

34. List four major causes of airway obstruction in the postoperative patient.

a.
b.
c.
d.

Circulation

35. List four areas to assess to determine a postoperative patient's circulatory status.

a.
b.
c.
d.

36. Describe the characteristic findings associated with postoperative hemorrhage.

a. Blood pressure:

b. Heart rate and character of pulse:

c. Respiratory rate:

d. Skin:

e. Level of consciousness:

Temperature control

37. Explain why patients awakening from surgery often complain of feeling cold.

38. Define *malignant hyperthermia.*

Copyright © 2019 Elsevier Canada, a division of Reed Elsevier Canada, Ltd.

Fluid and electrolyte balance

39. List three areas you should assess to determine fluid and electrolyte alterations.

    a. ______

    b. ______

    c. ______

Neurologic functions

40. List the areas of assessment that help to determine a postoperative patient's neurologic status.

    a. ______

    b. ______

    c. ______

    d. ______

Skin integrity and condition of the wound

41. The nurse assesses the condition of the skin, noting ______, ______, ______, and ______.

42. Describe how the nurse would assess the amount of drainage from a wound.

Genitourinary function

Depending on the surgery, a patient may not regain voluntary control over urinary function for 6 to 8 hours after anaesthesia.

Gastrointestinal function

43. Distension may occur in the patient who develops a ______.

44. Normally during the immediate recovery phase, faint or absent bowel sounds are auscultated in all four quadrants. Routinely, you auscultate the abdomen to detect return of normal bowel sounds; ______ loud gurgles per minute over each quadrant indicate that peristalsis has returned.

Pain and comfort

45. Pain can be perceived before full consciousness is regained. Acute incisional pain causes patients to become ______ and may be responsible for temporary changes in ______.

Assessment of the patient's discomfort and evaluation of pain relief therapies are essential nursing functions.

Nursing Diagnosis

46. Identify two actual or potential nursing diagnoses that are appropriate for a postoperative patient.

    a. ______

    b. ______

Planning

47. List the typical postoperative plans prescribed by surgeons and seen, for example, on clinical pathways.

    a. ______

    b. ______

    c. ______

    d. ______

    e. ______

    f. ______

    g. ______

    h. ______

    i. ______

    j. ______

    k. ______

Goals and outcomes

48. Give five goals of care and associated outcomes for a postoperative patient.

    a. ______

    b. ______

    c. ______

    d. ______

    e. ______

Implementation

Health promotion

49. To prevent respiratory complications, begin pulmonary interventions early. Describe measures that will promote the following:

    a. Airway patency:

    b. Expansion of the lungs:

Copyright © 2019 Elsevier Canada, a division of Reed Elsevier Canada, Ltd.

c. Removal of pulmonary secretions:

Preventing Circulatory Complications

50. Briefly describe measures to promote normal venous return and circulatory blood flow.
    a.
    b.
    c.
    d.
    e.
    f.

Achieving Rest and Comfort

51. List three nonpharmacologic pain-relief measures.
    a.
    b.
    c.

Acute care

52. Identify two postoperative nursing interventions for the following:
    a. Temperature regulation:
    b. Maintaining neurologic function:
    c. Maintaining fluid and electrolyte balances:
    d. Promoting normal bowel elimination and adequate nutrition:
    e. Promoting urinary elimination:
    f. Promoting wound healing:
    g. Maintaining and enhancing self-concept:

Evaluation

Patient care

The nurse evaluates the effectiveness of care provided to the surgical patient on the basis of expected outcomes following nursing interventions.

53. Describe how you should evaluate the ambulatory surgical patient.

REVIEW QUESTIONS

Select the appropriate answer, and cite the rationale for choosing that particular answer.

1. Mrs. Yong-Hing, a 45-year-old patient with diabetes, is having a hysterectomy in the morning. What would the nurse expect, given the patient's history?
   a. An increased risk of hemorrhaging
   b. Fluid imbalances
   c. Altered elimination of anaesthetic agents
   d. Impaired wound healing

Answer: ______ Rationale: ______

2. Which of the following is *not* included in the health history for the patient who is to have surgery?
   a. Identifying the patient's perception about surgery
   b. Obtaining information about the patient's past experience with surgery
   c. Deciding whether surgery is indicated
   d. Understanding the impact surgery has on the patient's and family's emotional health

Answer: ______ Rationale: ______

Copyright © 2019 Elsevier Canada, a division of Reed Elsevier Canada, Ltd.

3. Which of the following patients is *not* at risk for developing serious fluid and electrolyte imbalances during and after surgery?
   a. Patient E, who is 81 years old and is having emergency surgery for a bowel obstruction following 4 days of vomiting and diarrhea
   b. Patient F, who is 1 year old and is having a cleft palate repair
   c. Patient G, who is 55 years old and has a history of chronic respiratory disease
   d. Patient H, who is 79 years old and has a history of congestive heart failure

Answer: ______________ Rationale: ____________

____

____

4. What is the primary purpose of postoperative leg exercises?
   a. Promote venous return
   b. Promote lymphatic drainage
   c. Assess range of motion
   d. Exercise fatigued muscles

Answer: ______________ Rationale: ____________

____

____

5. The PACU nurse notices that the patient is shivering. What is the most common cause of this?
   a. The use of a reflective blanket on the OR table
   b. Side effects of certain anaesthetic agents
   c. IV narcotics used for pain management
   d. Malignant hypothermia

Answer: ______________ Rationale: ____________

____

____

CRITICAL THINKING MODEL FOR NURSING CARE PLAN FOR DEFICIENT KNOWLEDGE REGARDING PREOPERATIVE AND POSTOPERATIVE CARE REQUIREMENTS

Imagine that you are Joe, the nurse in the Care Plan on pages 1377–1378 of your text. Complete the *evaluation* phase of the critical thinking model by writing your answers in the appropriate boxes of the model shown. Think about the following:

- During evaluation, what knowledge and professional standards were applied to Mrs. Campana's care?
- In what way might Joe's previous experience influence his evaluation of Mrs. Campana's care?
- In what way do critical thinking attitudes play a role in how you approach the evaluation of Mrs. Campana's care plan?
- How might Joe adjust Mrs. Campana's care?
- What knowledge did Joe apply in evaluating Mrs. Campana's care?

Copyright © 2019 Elsevier Canada, a division of Reed Elsevier Canada, Ltd.

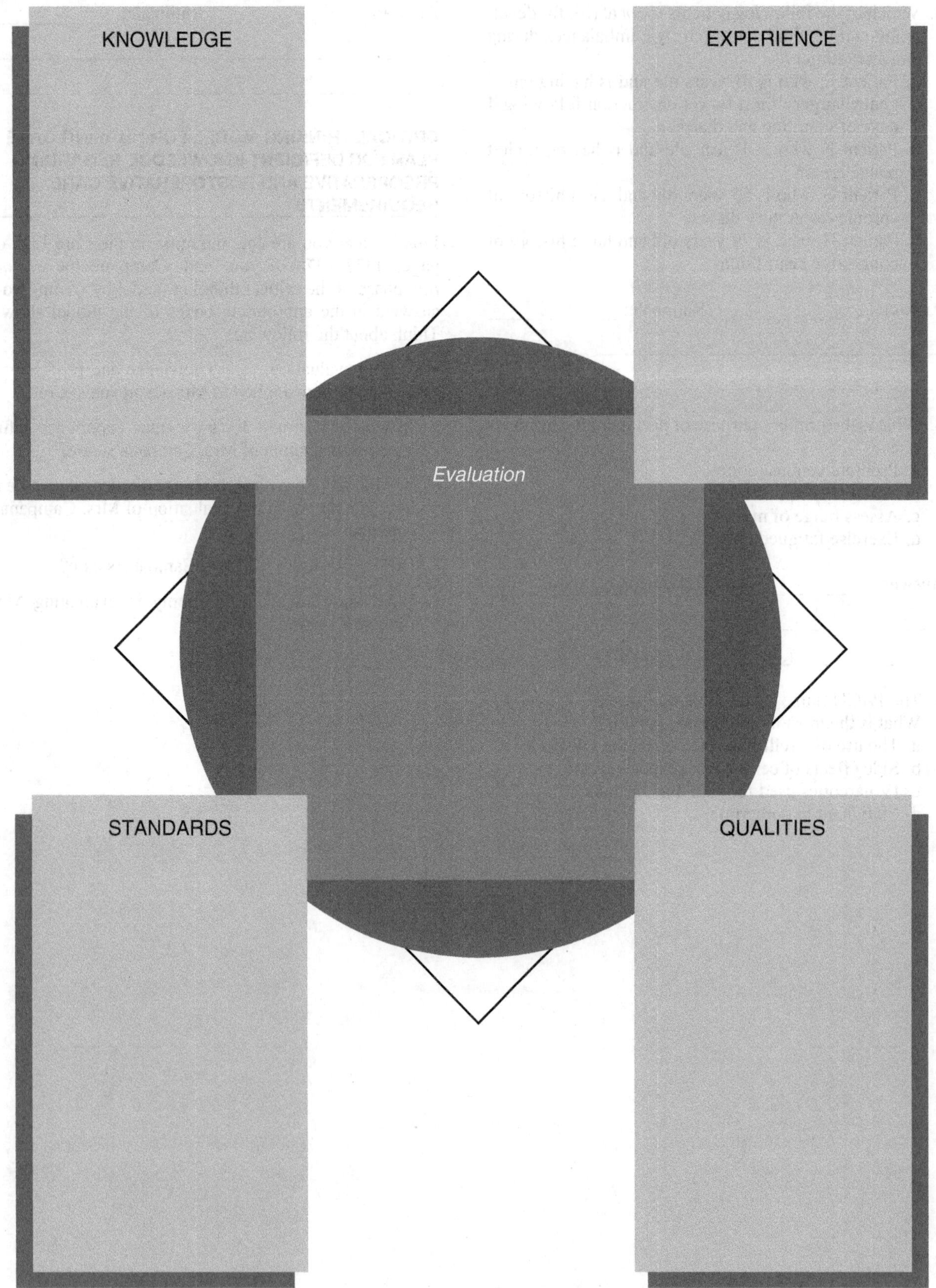

CHAPTER 48 Critical Thinking Model for Nursing Care Plan for *Deficient Knowledge Regarding Preoperative and Postoperative Care Requirements*

See answers on Evolve site.

Copyright © 2019 Elsevier Canada, a division of Reed Elsevier Canada, Ltd.